COMMUNITY HEALTH NEEDS ASSESSMENT

COMMUNITY HEALTH NEEDS ASSESSMENT

The Healthcare Professional's Guide to Evaluating the Needs in Your Defined Market

Timothy W. Bosworth

A Healthcare 2000 Publication

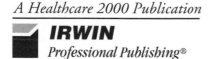
IRWIN
Professional Publishing®

Chicago • London • Singapore

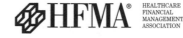
HEALTHCARE
FINANCIAL
MANAGEMENT
ASSOCIATION

A Healthcare 2000 Publication

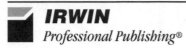

IRWIN
Professional Publishing®

© Richard D. Irwin, a Times Mirror Higher Education Group, Inc. company, 1996

This publication is designed to provide accurate and authoritative information in regard to the subject matter covered. It is sold with the understanding that neither the author nor the publisher is engaged in rendering legal, accounting, or other professional service. If legal advice or other expert assistance is required, the services of a competent professional person should be sought.

From a Declaration of Principles jointly adopted by a Committee of the American Bar Association and a Committee of Publishers.

Irwin Professional Book Team

Publisher: *Wayne McGuirt*
Associate publisher: *Jim McNeil*
Sponsoring editor: *Kristine Rynne*
Marketing manager: *Cindy L. Ledwith*
Project editor: *Christina Thornton-Villagomez*
Production supervisor: *Dina L. Tredaway*
Assistant manager, desktop services: *Jon Christopher*
Designer: *L. Cope*
Compositor: *ZGraphics, Ltd.*
Typeface: *11/13 Times Roman*
Printer: *Buxton Skinner*

Times Mirror
M Higher Education Group

Library of Congress Cataloging-in-Publication Data

Bosworth, Timothy W.
     Community health needs assessment / Timothy W. Bosworth.
          p.   cm.
     "Healthcare 2000 publication."
     ISBN 1–55738–647–1
     1. Hospitals—Health promotion services—United States—Planning.
 2. Community health services—United States—Evaluation. 3. Medical
 care—Needs assessment—United States. I. Title.
 RA975.5.H4B67   1996
 362.1'2'0973—dc20   95–36932

Printed in the United States of America
1 2 3 4 5 6 7 8 9 0 BS 2 1 0 9 8 7 6 5

Contents

Acknowledgments

A number of people have helped make this book possible. First, I wish to thank my clients, whose data are used in this book. Without their involvement, I would not have entered the area of community health needs assessment at all. Second, I wish to thank the president and staff of Young & Associates, Inc., in Kent, Ohio, whose support and tolerance enabled me to work in this area. Third, I wish to thank my publisher, Richard D. Irwin, Inc., who responded with interest in publishing a book about this area of health needs. Above all, I would like to thank my wife, Deborah Cole, who somehow managed to put up with my maniacal single-mindedness and whose generous love and support make everything more meaningful.

Timothy W. Bosworth

Chapter One

The Argument

In Wisconsin, they tell this story. Imagine that you are sitting outside your home on the bank of a swiftly flowing river. Suddenly, you see a man struggling in the current. You swim to the man and pull him out of the river. He thanks you, gives you $20 out of gratitude, and goes on his way. The next day, you see a woman struggling downstream. You rescue her, she thanks you, gives you $20 out of gratitude, and goes on her way. From then on, each day more people float downstream in need of rescue, and you become very adept at rescuing them. In fact, the supply of struggling people becomes so great that you organize a rescue organization, operating out of your house. Your reputation has grown, and the community has provided funding to support your valuable community service. You do a good job, add a lot of staff, and invest heavily in expensive equipment, and you can boast that you have never allowed anyone to drown—except a few who were nearly dead when you reached them.

One day a stranger from another country visits the town. He has heard about your rescue service, become intrigued, and has come to learn more about it. You show him around, and he is impressed. In fact, while he is there, you successfully rescue several more people. Being from out of town, he doesn't know the history of your organization, and he doesn't share the adoration of the community. He then asks why all these people are falling in the river in the first place. You shrug your shoulders, and he innocently asks the following question: "Wouldn't it be a good idea for you to examine the river upstream to find out why so many people are falling into the river in the first place and why they have such trouble swimming?" You reply that it is a good question. But you are really too busy with operational issues, you don't have the time, you can't free any of your staff to do it, and maybe you can get to it in a few months after you have gotten ready for the state rescue commission's visit.

Chief executive officers of America's hospitals are a little like the "you" in this parable, and I am a little like the man who visited from another country. In the past, it was assumed that hospitals had to be responsible only for those people who entered their buildings, under the assumption that a hospital's responsibility extended no farther than the exit lamp. Hospitals built successful operations and heavily invested in staff and other resources in the rescuing. But, a few years ago, we passed through a door, labeled "new paradigm," and entered an arena of altered expectations. Passing through this door signaled a number of parallel shifts: from a medical model that favors treatment of disease, illness, and medical maladies to wellness, focusing on health, quality of life, and health promotion; from a stress on high technology intervention to low technology prevention; from seeing patients as customers to seeing communities as customers; from a competitive model to a collaborative model; from reactive thinking to proactive thinking; from fragmented medical services to integrated systems; and from seeing the hospital as a repair shop to the hospital as a catalyst for promoting healthful living.

More often than before, a healthcare provider is expected to be responsible for maintaining and improving the health of all people in the community, under the assumption that chief executive officers should spend some time looking upstream to examine the sources of their business and to explore ways of doing business differently. In fact, in the very near future, if not now, you will be asked to assume responsibility for the health of the communities you serve. If you share the responsibility for that care with other providers, all of you will need to find ways to work together for the common good. Providing technically excellent medical care inside your building is no longer good enough.

Satisfying these new assumptions begins with a community health needs assessment, the subject of this book. This is a large undertaking. You will have to address a number of issues. What community does your hospital serve? How should you study it? Should you work alone or together with other providers? What do you do with information after you get it? Should you involve an outside firm? Which of your staff should you involve? These are some of the issues addressed in this book.

The argument of this book is this: (1) Hospitals already have within their mission improving the health of patients. It is not, therefore, a large leap to argue that hospitals should forge new roles for themselves as catalysts of healthier communities. You should take on yourself the primary role in conducting community health needs assessments and of developing plans to improve the health status of the community. (2) You should attempt to create a communitywide effort to develop the project. You should not work on your own, unless others do not follow your lead. But, even if others do not follow your lead, you should push ahead. I believe that, once the community sees that your hospital is working earnestly and is inviting its participation, the community will respond. (3) The assessment process should begin with a study. It should rely on a mix of quantitative and qualitative data, and it should take in a range of different kinds of sources of information. It should be comprehensive, well-designed, well-thought-out, carefully prepared, and responsive to the wishes and demands of the community. (4) You should involve an independent research team or a private research firm to conduct the research and render its independent opinion of the results. You should also be closely involved in the project. (5) You should then use the study as a springboard toward ongoing community health needs assessment. (6) You should not allow the study to gather dust on the shelf. If you do, you have done little to improve the health of the community and have only supported the research team's lifestyle.

Obviously, there are other points of view on this subject. Some argue that the local health departments should take the lead. Others argue that the communities themselves should be the sparkplug. I do not disagree with any of these other points of view. If you are approached by a community group or by a local health department, by all means get involved in its process. Do not try to arm wrestle with it. However, be an active participant. You will find, as many before you have found, that the process is an effective planning tool. After all, your hospital's goal is to determine the need for your products and services, and community health needs assessment is an important first step. This book can help you get started in the process and give you things to think about while you are in it. If you just want to learn about the process, this book can help you do that. If you are involved in the process and want another slant, this book will help you do that, too.

Now, for what this book is *not*. First, it is not about health promotion; it is a book about health assessment. Health promotion involves a range of activities and initiatives related to studying the health of the community, to designing strategies for implementing those strategies, to advocating healthy behaviors, and to evaluating the effort. Community health needs assessment is only the first part of the overall health promotion process. Second, this book is not a workbook to show you how to do the assessment. There are plenty of such books on the market. I review a number of them in this book, and if you are interested in them after reading this book, you should look for one of those books. Third, it is not a research methods textbook. It will not tell you everything about how to do research. There are shelves and shelves of methods textbooks out there.

This book is written for three audiences. First, those who have heard about community health needs assessment—or who have a passing interest in it and want to find out more about it—can find out about this area of inquiry. Second, those who are involved in community health needs assessment can read a different perspective. He or she may agree or disagree with me, but I am convinced that my argument has merit, and I am presumptive enough to believe firmly that another point of view can be helpful. Third, the book can benefit those who have been asked to conduct a needs assessment; they can gain some pointers from this book. From this book, you will learn the following: what community assessment is; why people do community health needs assessment; how it is accomplished; what its basic components are; what you can find out from the process; what models are available for your use; what you can learn from it about your community; what is going on in the area of community health needs assessment.

I write this book as a research professional with practical experience both in the healthcare field and in community development and neighborhood action. While completing my graduate work at the University of Wisconsin, I purchased a house in a part of Madison referred to as South Madison, a special needs area of the city with a concentrated minority population and a number of public housing complexes. While the few blocks around my house were quite safe, other areas were experiencing nascent gang development, poverty, unemployment, discrimination, and, though on a smaller scale, many of the urban problems that confront many American cities. I became president of the South Madison Neighborhood Center and helped found the South Madison Community Development Corporation and the South Madison Business Association. In my role as president of the center, I was involved in some early needs assessment conducted by the center's parent corporation. As a market research professional, I often have been called on to help hospitals understand how they can compete more effectively with other hospitals. Because of my community involvement and my professional training, community health needs assessment is for me an important answer for hospitals and communities to work together to improve the conditions under which people live.

HEALTH NEEDS ASSESSMENT IN AMERICA

Health needs assessment has grown from a trickle a few years ago to a flood. In some places hospitals are leading the effort, in other places the local health departments are leading the effort, and in still other places community groups have taken the initiative. There are no instruments capable of measuring precisely the dimensions of the flow, but my review suggests that it is close to a social movement—an uneven social movement, but a social movement nonetheless.

Some examples suggest the ubiquity of efforts. These are but four examples of health promotion efforts across the country of which health assessment is a cornerstone.

Waukesha, Wisconsin

In November 1993, Waukesha County, Wisconsin, together with the State of Wisconsin Division of Health and area healthcare facilities, came together to develop an assessment and health promotion effort. The county executive appointed a Healthy Waukesha 2000 Committee, which analyzed health information and held communitywide forums. Eight work groups developed goals and actions, which became key elements in a resulting plan. The plan specified goals and objectives, identified community organizations that can help in the process, and identified strategies for improvement of the health status of Waukesha County.

Baltimore, Maryland

Baltimore is highly urbanized and mostly African-American—and is plagued by rising mortality and morbidity, unemployment, crime, substandard housing, and a deficient educational system. A health promotion effort, called "Heart, Body, and Soul Program," worked through a coalition of community organizations, agencies, businesses, and healthcare providers to establish prevention centers and training programs to focus on reducing the effects of smoking, hypertension, diabetes, tuberculosis, cancer, and coronary disease. The organization has established community crime patrols, crime prevention education workshops, housing, education, and economic development programs.

Dalton, Georgia

A high prevalence of high school dropouts, drunk-driving convictions, and medical indigence mobilized a coalition of more than 100 physicians, hospital executives, government officials, educators, social service directors, business executives, and minority leaders to assess the region's health and social problems and develop action plans. Results included a health center pilot project for three elementary schools, a comprehensive health course for 10 third grade classes, and expanded indigent care services. A healthcare financing mechanism for small employers is under study, and literacy and consumer health education groups are being formed.

Wray, Colorado

This community numbers 1,998 people and has dedicated itself to improving community health through prevention and intervention. The showpiece of Wray's efforts is a rehabilitation and activities center—a fitness and healthy lifestyle center for all residents, including senior citizens, who previously lacked such a resource. The prevention-based Family Center offers classes on social, family, and individual issues, all designed to help avoid serious family crises.

Why Should You Invest in a Community Health Needs Assessment?

Should you invest in community health needs assessments? I have listed six questions. Take time now to answer each one.

1. Has your hospital lost the trust of your community? Do you think your hospital is viewed as an institution "that wishes to do well rather than do good?" A recent survey, quoted in the Wisconsin Hospital Association's guide, found that "approximately two-thirds of people surveyed saw hospitals as business enterprises rather than as social service organizations, and that almost half should pay taxes."[1] From now on, an important indicator of your hospital's success may well be the overall health of the community you serve.

2. Are the people or organizations that pay your bills, requiring or will they soon require, your hospital to meet certain population-based quality and performance standards, or is it likely that in the future they will do so?

This trend is growing, illustrated by the increased usage of report cards and epidemiological indicators regarding community health.

3. Is capitation in or nearing your community? It has begun where providers receive a fixed payment to care for the health of a defined population. This lends a powerful incentive for promoting the health of the community.

4. Is your hospital required by a federal or state government or agency to conduct a community health needs assessment? In New York, Indiana, and Texas, many hospitals are required to conduct community health needs assessments and to submit yearly plans.

5. Do you think you might face a potential public relations nightmare without doing one? Would you be surprised if a reporter from your local newspaper walked into your office tomorrow and asked to see your community service plan, even if there is no legal requirement for you to provide one, and then wrote an article criticizing your hospital?

6. Do you think that looking upstream to find ways to improve the health of your community is the right thing to do? Do you want a sound planning process that will help you do your job better?

If you have already undertaken an assessment for one or more of the reasons listed, you have already answered one or more of these questions. But if you have not, and you have registered a "yes" or "not sure," you may well wish to get started right away. If you have answered "no" on all the questions, you may wish to do some personal strategic planning.

NOW WHAT ARE WE TALKING ABOUT?

The concept of community health needs assessment as a field of inquiry has four components: "community," "health," "needs," and "assessment." Before proceeding further in this book, it will be important to think about what these concepts mean.[2]

Community

Turning first to the notion of "community," we usually find an implication of commonness attributed to a group of people who share common interests, characteristics, and a common fate in the world. Webster gives us the following as synonyms: aggregation, association, commonwealth, society, order, class, brotherhood, fraternity, polity, unity, nationality, similarity.

Webster gives as the first meaning the "common possession or enjoyment; as a **community** of goods," as in the English philosopher John Locke's reference to "the original **community** of all things." Webster continues: "a society of people having common rights and privileges, or common interests, civil, political, or ecclesiastical, or living under the same laws and regulations; as a **community** of farmers." Webster lists, as a third definition, the "society at large; the public, or people in general; in this sense used with the definite article; as, burdens laid upon the poor classes of **the community**;" and a fourth definition of community as "a common character; similarity; likeness; as, **community** of spirit," referring to Herbert Spencer's line referring to "the essential **community** of nature between organic growth and inorganic growth." Finally, Webster lists several more "down to earth" concepts of community: "the district, city, etc., where [people] live."[3]

Health

We find embedded in the concept of health the quality of being sound in mind, body, and spirit, of being wholesome, robust, hale, and vigorous. Webster defines health primarily as the "physical and mental well-being; soundness; freedom from defect, pain, or disease; normality of mental and physical functions," and as a "condition of body or mind; as good or bad **health**." We also find in Webster two more unusual meanings of health: (1) the "power to heal, restore, or purify," as summarized in the proverb "the tongue of the wise is **health**"; and (2) "a toast wishing health and wellness to another; as, to drink one's **health**," as excerpted in the Shakespearean line, "come, love and **health**."[4]

Needs

Embedded in the definition of needs is the twin concept of a lack or a limitation of something required, and a call to action to correct the deficiency or to supply something to fill a gap. These can be inferred from the following synonyms given by Webster: exigency, emergency, strait, extremity, necessity, distress, destitution, poverty, indigence, and penury. Specifically, Webster gives four definitions of "need": (1) "a necessity; compulsion, obligation; as, there is no **need** to worry now"; "a lack of something useful, required, or desired; a call or demand for the presence, possession, etc. of something; as, I feel the **need** of a long rest"; (2)

"something useful, required, or desired that is lacking; want; requirements; as, what are his daily **needs**?"; (3) "a condition in which there is a deficiency of something; a time or situation of difficulty; a condition requiring relief or supply; as, a friend in **need**"; and (4) "a condition of poverty; state of extreme want; as **if need be**; if it is required; if the occasion demands; or **to have need to**; to be compelled or required to; must."⁵

Assessment

In analyzing the concept of "assessment," we find that recent usage has departed considerably from the strict definition of the word. Webster tells us that to assess is to "set or fix a certain sum against, as a tax, fine, or special payment; as, to **assess** each citizen in due proportion; also, to impose (a certain amount) as a tax, fine, etc." A further definition of "to assess" is the following: "to fix the value of (property) for the purposes of being taxed," or "to set the amount of (damages, a fine, etc.)." Going on, an assessment is "an assessing; specifically a valuation of property for the purpose of taxation." Webster also defines it as "a method or schedule of assessing, or an amount assessed." A final definition, under Webster, is: "*(a)* payment asked on a stock subscription, usually at stated intervals," or "*(b)* a levy for political purposes, called a **political assessment.**"

What we mean by the term *to assess* is closer to the third meaning of assessment, "evaluation" or appraisal. But it comes closer to the meaning of the term *to investigate*: "to trace out, search into; to inquire into systematically; to examine in detail with care and accuracy; as, to **investigate** the powers and forces of nature; to **investigate** the conduct of an agent." And what we mean by an assessment is closer to the meaning of investigation: "careful search; detailed examination; systematic inquiry; as, the **investigations** of the scientist; the **investigations** of the district attorney."⁶

At the risk of being overly etymological, the concept of assessment, as we use it, involves what Webster defines as analysis: the separating or breaking up of any whole "into its parts so as to find out their nature, proportion, function, relationship, etc.," or "the examination of the constituents or parts of; determine the nature of tendencies of," and "analysis," which is defined as "a statement of the results of this process."⁷

This inquiry shows that, when we say we are assessing the needs of a community, we are not being precise, because we are not really placing a value on needs for purposes of taxation. We are really investigating, rather than assessing. Even though it isn't precise, we had better follow the usage, anyway, because we are like a man walking an elephant on a leash—if the elephant wants to go somewhere, we'd best tag along.

Putting It All Together

Having examined each component together gives us a basis for proceeding. Community health needs assessment, for the purposes of this book, refers to an investigation to find out what is lacking in the physical, social, psychological, and environmental makeup of the area in which people who have a common interest live, to determine what should be done to improve the physical, social, psychological, and environmental conditions under which residents of that area live.

I mean by community health needs assessment something different from what others think it means. To many, the assessment process includes assessing the health status of a community, exciting the community to action, and assessing the process. I see this process as health promotion, of which health needs assessment is only the first step. While I am on the subject, community health needs assessment differs from community benefit analysis. Community benefit analysis involves quantifying the benefit of the hospital to the community. It is a parallel activity but not the same as health needs assessment.

NEEDS AND WANTS

An important distinction to be made at the outset is between needs and wants. Turning again to Webster, we see that *want* means "to desire; to wish; as, she wants to go with us," and, alternatively, "to feel a desire for, as for something absent, needed, lost, or the like; to feel the need of; to wish or long for; to desire; to crave."[8] Whereas a *need* involves a requirement or obligation, a *want* involves a perception or a perceived need. A "need" is something observed objectively by another toward the person who needs; a "want" is something generated internally and is best judged by the person.

Now, let me explain what I see as a major area of confusion in needs investigation. Most people don't have a very clear understanding of what their own needs are. They can only know their wants. When my teenage son comes to me and says, "Dad, I need a car," he is telling me not what his "need" is but what his want is. He wants a car because his friends have them, he would like to feel grown-up, or he wants to be liked by his friends. He wants a car, but he doesn't need one, notwithstanding the fact that everyone he knows also lives on the same block, that he lives across the street from the school and has a job on the next street. However, if on graduation, he comes to me and tells me, "Dad, I have an interview with Aardvark Corporation scheduled for next week," I may then respond: "Oh, gee, that's great, son. You will need a suit." Then we have determined what his need is. Of course, if he doesn't really have to work and he doesn't really need the job but only wants the job to give himself a feeling of self-worth, that is another question. This distinction is a key one, yet it is violated all the time. It may seem obvious, but it will be important to keep this distinction in mind as we discuss some of the methodological implications of community health needs investigation.

WHAT YOU WILL LEARN FROM AN ASSESSMENT

Conducting a community health needs assessment is a little like finding your way at a service station. Many of us travel. At some point in our travels, almost every one of us has looked around and asked where we are. Recently, I took a trip to San Diego, California. My wife and I were driving through La Jolla. There is a beautiful park down by the sea that features some steep-sided cliffs where many birds "hang out" for rest and relaxation. Wanting to do some serious bird watching, we were looking for a narrow road that led down to the park, but we were having trouble finding the right one. I had a good map with me, but it wasn't helping because I didn't know where I was. I tried to find my way for a while, but I soon realized that, at the rate I was going, it would be quite late at night before I found the park, if I ever did, because I was lost. So, I pulled into a service station and asked were we were. The attendant showed me that I was about two miles beyond the park, driving in the wrong direction. I turned around and, in a few minutes, my wife and I found ourselves happily faced with hundreds of interesting birds. Well, conducting community health assessments is a little like this. If you are just starting out, it gives you a starting point. If you are along the way, it helps you to evaluate your progress and measure your distance from your ultimate goal. If you have reached your goal, an assessment will show you other routes. I see an assessment report as the first piece of the puzzle. It incorporates a range of research results, which allow one to chart one's course along the road fueled with sound strategies. A sound assessment should have five elements: (1) an assessment plan, (2) a community profile, (3) a determination of the key health needs of the community, (4) estimates of the health status of the community, and (5) recommendations for action.

Assessment Plan

The first step in any assessment is devising an assessment plan. This is a very brief document, similar to a marketing plan for business. It lays out the reasons for doing what you are doing, what the goals and objectives of the effort are, when you envision achieving them, how you are going to reach them, and how you will evaluate your progress. The plan should be just detailed enough to give you guidance, but it will be revised several times during the course of the health promotion process. The plan should also specify your strategy for developing community support and involvement of the community.

Community Profile

The second step involves developing a community profile. This profile is developed from a number of sources: census data, county health departments, hospital discharge inventories, research reports from private or public agencies and organizations, and other sources. Census data are available in most public libraries, university archives, and governmental planning offices. Most state universities have people trained in using the census and other federal data documents and are anxious to provide to users any information at their command. This profile is important to help the investigator gain an eye on the community and to assemble all that is currently known about the health status of the community.

Needs Analysis

Third, one must identify and document the key health problems in the community and specify underserved groups. No matter where you are, some group is underserved. If you are in a large, densely settled urban area, inner-city minority groups will be underserved. If you are in a sparsely settled rural area, the primary underserved group will be rural poor. If you are in a agricultural area, migrant workers might be an underserved group. If you are in an area that has experienced the stresses of in-migration, undocumented migrants may be a key group. These groups are not very accessible to you and are the most suspicious of you, yet they are the most vulnerable. They have a lower than average ability to access the medical service delivery system, yet they have the greatest need. The question becomes, then, "How does one find out what their needs are when one can't reach them?"

Answering this question is not as difficult as it first seems To assess their needs, you don't have to reach them. In fact, as we discussed earlier in this chapter, it wouldn't help you if you did. They won't talk to you, and they can't tell you what they need, anyway. They can only tell you what they want. I don't mean to say we shouldn't pay any attention to what they want, I only argue that we should keep that in perspective, just as I keep my son's expressed desire for his own car in perspective. A teenager doesn't need a car like he needs food. And it is a good thing, too, considering how much a teenager eats. So, to get back on track, the second element in an assessment is a needs analysis.

Interviewing community stakeholders will pinpoint efficiently and effectively the most pressing health needs of the community. People know of only what they want; stakeholders know what they need. Community stakeholders include the following: government leaders, business executives, public health officials, chamber of commerce representatives, social service agency representatives, service club presidents, local college or university faculty and administrators, physicians, hospital employees, union leaders, and anyone else who is active in meeting social needs in your community. I always include social service representatives and then work in other types of community leaders as appropriate. You will see how this works in the next series of chapters. I favor using an expanded definition of health, one that incorporates the social, psychological, emotional, spiritual, and environmental well-being in addition to freedom from diseases.

Here are some of the needs we have identified in different areas through this phase of the assessment process: decreased child and domestic abuse, fewer teenage pregnancies and better prenatal care, more widely available or less expensive health insurance, a better transportation system, a more reliable ambulance service, more doctors or specialists, better coordination among social service providers, more comprehensive services for the elderly, and less alcohol and drug abuse. The community leader survey will also enable you to build support for health improvement efforts. Once leaders have identified a key need, you can ask them whether or not they would be willing to assist in working with the community to address the problem. If they say yes, and most will, you have developed a basis for increased collaboration with those leaders' organizations.

Health-Related Behavior Survey

A fourth element in my community health needs assessment is a survey of health-related behaviors. Data from this survey will be used to develop health status indicators, those factors shown by research to affect, positively or negatively, the health of a community. Health status indicators measure the prevalence of the following: use of safety belts, high blood pressure, consumption of alcohol and other drugs, driving while drunk, cancer, diabetes, obesity, lack of regular exercise, utilization of medical facilities, and other behaviors that affect the health of the community.

This part of the assessment embodies the results of a survey of households in the community, selected randomly throughout the community. The sample size will depend on the complexity of your community, the desired power of the analysis, and the uses to which the data will be put. In some areas, 200 interviews may be sufficient; in others, 1,000 interviews may be required. Taken from the Behavioral Risk Factor Surveillance System questionnaire, developed by the Centers for Disease Control and Prevention, it questions people about behaviors, from calories consumed to cancer screening, to measure community health status. The CDC survey is conducted on a monthly basis in each state. Most surveys collect the same data using the same questionnaire, though some states add extra "modules," or groups of questions. Data for your state are probably available through your department or division of health, but may not be county specific. Collecting comparable data for the communities of interest allows comparison with the local data, where available, with the state data, where feasible, and with public service goals given in *Healthy People 2000*.

Comparing data is important. For example, if the prevalence of smoking in your area is 32 percent, and the comparable rate of smoking for the state as a whole is 32 percent, it is clear that the community is probably typical of the state as a whole, and that probably if you work at it you won't change the behavior much. However, if you know that the prevalence of smoking in your community is 55 percent, but 28 percent for the state, it is clear that the community is markedly higher than the statewide average with respect to that behavior, and you may be able to effect a greater change by focusing more resources on it. This gives you a reasonable way of developing targets and strategies. Comparing data against public health goals gives you other targets. The public health service goal for smoking is the reduction to 15 percent among adults 20 or older. If the proportion of smokers in your area is 55 percent, you know that you have your work cut out for you. If the proportion of smokers in your area is 16 percent, then you may find that another goal may be more important.

Preparing a Report with Recommended Actions

The final component of a health needs assessment is translating problems into action. Reviewing the research results and establishing priorities for action constitute the final component. You should select one to five issues for action, and concentrate only on one or two of the most pressing issues. Your assessment plan should specify your next steps and how you are going to implement the findings. You should then review your plan in light of the research results, taking into account any relevant events that may have occurred in your community since you wrote the preliminary plan. With these documents in hand, the assessment process is complete, and you can do the really hard part—acting to improve the health of the community.

Some Distinctions

Let me repeat my discussion of how my notion of community health needs assessment differs from the notions of others. Others see the process as an ongoing process, running from beginning to end, from summoning a community task force to collecting and analyzing data, devising objectives, writing plans, implementing plans, and assessing the process and results. My view of community health needs assessment involves only the first portion of this effort. I see it as essentially a research process, focusing on collecting information and assisting with the development of implementation strategies and plans. The rest of it is important but lies in health promotion efforts, not assessment.

Another distinction to be made is between community benefit analysis and community health needs assessments. Community benefit analysis refers to the process of identifying and quantifying the value of the different ways in which the hospital benefits the community. Valuing charity care, for example, is part of the community benefit analysis process.

TO SUM UP

Thus, my approach incorporates five elements: developing an assessment plan, drawing a community profile, conducting a community leader survey, surveying behaviors related to the health of communities, and preparing a report that ranks problems in the order they should be addressed. In the following chapters, we examine the fruits of this approach in several areas of the country: central Missouri, central California, northern Missouri, central Iowa, and northern Indiana.

The plan of the book is as follows. Chapters One through Six present case studies showing the results we have achieved based on the process I use. Then, for those of you who want to read about other ways of doing community health needs assessments, Chapter Seven reviews eight different approaches to community health needs assessment. Then, Chapter Eight argues that you should involve an independent research team to conduct your research. But, Bosworth be damned, in case you disagree with my reasoning and wish to do your own anyway, I offer some tips on the most commonly used research methods. Then, Chapter Nine offers, as a kind of going-away present, an overview of community health needs assessment initiatives and activities in most of the states. Chapter Ten offers some concluding thoughts.

ENDNOTES

1. American Hospital Association. *Community Benefit and Tax Exempt Status: A Self Assessment Guide for Hospitals*, p. 1; quoted in *Collaboration for Health; a Guide to Building Healthier Communities*. Madison: Wisconsin Hospital Association, 1995, p. 11.
2. *Webster's New Twentieth Century Dictionary of the English Language, Unabridged*. 2d ed. Edited by Jean L. McKechnie. Cleveland: World Publishing Company, 1963.

3. Webster, p. 367.
4. Webster, p. 836.
5. Webster, p. 1201.
6. Webster, p. 966.
7. Webster, pp. 64 and 65.
8. Webster, p. 2059.

Chapter Two

Central Missouri

OVERVIEW

This chapter summarizes the results of a study conducted in central Missouri during the summer of 1994. The study consisted of four components: first, a review of selected information from the 1990 federal census identified key demographic characteristics of the three-county area; second, a special survey of community leaders and social service agency representatives determined the most pressing health issues, problems, or concerns in each of the three counties; third, results from a survey of the community sampled the public's opinion concerning the local hospital and described the health status of the community; and, finally, a fourth component examined discharges from the hospital to calculate the percentage of conditions that were preventable. In reporting the results, I have changed the names of the counties and hospitals to protect the confidentiality of my clients.

PROFILE OF THE ASSESSMENT AREA

The assessment area included three counties, designated here as South, East, and North. They lie in central Missouri, roughly a 90-minute drive from each of three larger cities to the northeast, to the northwest, and to the south. A major highway connects the area with a large community to the northeast. The area is a major focus of recreation and retirement, and it attracts a large seasonal population as well as a growing elderly population. South County Hospital, located near the intersection of the three counties, is the only healthcare facility in the three-county area, but residents also seek care at larger tertiary hospitals in the larger cities.

The 1990 census lists 25,551 households in the tri-county area: 11,305 in South County, 7,977 in East County, and 6,269 in North County. The median age of people in the area assessed is considerably higher than the

state as a whole. The proportion of people aged 65 years or over is higher
than the statewide percentage, and a relatively low proportion of people
are under 45 years old. East and North counties have a relatively high proportion of elderly women living alone. In South County, the proportion
seems to be considerably lower. The area has a high proportion of high
school dropouts, a significantly lower proportion of persons aged 18 to 24
enrolled in college, and a significantly lower proportion of high school
graduates than the state as a whole. These counties have a high proportion
of families defined as poor. Median household income, measured in 1989,
is considerably lower than that for the state as a whole. Median household
size and the percentage of the labor force defined as unemployed vary by
county but are roughly the same as the statewide area. (See Exhibit 2–1.)

EXHIBIT 2–1
Population Characteristics by County

	County			
	South	*East*	*North*	*State*
Mean household size	2.41	2.56	2.44	2.54
Percent of women over 65 living alone	6.9	9.7	9.5	9.0
Age distribution:				
Under 5	5.8	7.4	6.6	7.2
Under 18	21.8	27.9	23.1	25.7
18 to 24	6.5	8.4	7.1	10.1
25 to 44	26.1	28.4	23.7	31.0
45 to 64	27.1	19.6	25.5	19.2
65 or over	18.4	15.5	20.6	14.0
80 or over	3.0	4.1	4.7	3.5
Median age	41.7	34.0	41.8	33.5
Percent persons aged 16–19 not enrolled in high school but not graduated	11.9	13.0	23.7	11.3
Percent persons aged 18 to 24 enrolled in college	16.0	11.0	12.3	34.3
Percent high school graduate or higher	73.0	63.0	64.3	73.9
Percent unemployed	5.8	7.2	6.2	6.2
Percent of families for whom poverty status is determined	10.2	13.6	12.0	10.1
Median household income	$22,564	$18,985	$19,158	$26,362

Source: U.S. Department of the Census, 1990: *Social and Economic Characteristics*, vol. CP-2-27,
Table 1 through Table 3; *General Population Statistics*, vol. CP-1-27, Tables 1 and 2.

Population projections supplied by the University of Missouri's Office of Social and Economic Data Analysis hold that, over the next 30 years, the proportion of Missouri's population over the age of 65 will grow 42 percent, and that the proportion of the population over age 85 will grow even faster. Though these projections are statewide, it is reasonable to assume that the elderly population in the three-county area studied here will grow even more rapidly than across the state, and that the youth population will continue to shrink.

HEALTH NEEDS: THE COMMUNITY LEADER PERSPECTIVE

A community leader survey pinpointed the primary health needs of the residents of East, North, and South counties. Health was broadly defined in line with the definition of health as noted in Chapter One. The analysis works from the assumption that a community hospital should work to provide maximum benefit by working to address the overall health of the community it serves. It sees medical implications of social problems and believes that, through action in the community to alleviate social problems, it can diminish the incidence of specific medical problems and improve the quality of life for all of the residents of the community.

The community leader survey covered the following areas: the most pressing health needs of the community, how well these problems are currently being addressed, and strategies that should be followed to make the greatest impact on the area's most pressing health problems. The reader should keep in mind that the analysis on which this part of the chapter is based relies on the informed perception of people who are knowledgeable of the needs of the community.

To complete the survey, we contacted and interviewed representatives of social service agencies, service clubs, governmental bodies, and the school system. To qualify for inclusion in our sample, agencies had to serve residents of the assessment area and had to be domiciled in it. Representatives of agencies based outside the three-county area were not interviewed.

Representatives of the following South County agencies and organizations were included in this survey: AR Funeral Home, South City Baptist Assembly, Bristol Manor, South City Chamber of Commerce, South City School District, South Senior Center, South County Commission, South County Family Services, South County Public Health Department, Mid-Missouri Ambulance District, chamber of commerce, South City administration, Springs City government, South City administration, State Division of Aging, Area Vocational–Technical School, South City Ambulance Service, Creek Village administration, South City Health Care Center, and the village administration of Beach, Missouri. Organizations based in East County included: East City Chamber of Commerce, East County Commission, East City government, East City Health Care Center, East City School District, East City administration, East County Division of Family Services, East County Ambulance Service, East County Funeral Home, and East County Public Health Department. Organizations based in North County included the North County Commission, the Commission on Aging, Shepherd Nursing Home, North County School District, North County Division of Family Services, North County Public Health Department, North Village administration, city government, and the North City Chamber of Commerce.

While reading the following, the reader should keep in mind that the quoted remarks reflect accurate paraphrases of respondents' remarks, rather than direct quotations.

We began the interview by pointing out that the purpose of our study was to "gain your perspective concerning the most important health issues or concerns in your county." After collecting some background information, we began by asking respondents the following question: "We're interested in your perspective as a person who is active in the affairs of your county, and we are looking at health in a very broad context, one that incorporates environmental, emotional, and psychological well-being in addition to the absence of disease. From this perspective, then, what would you say is the most pressing health problem, issue, or concern in the county right now?" Respondents were left to answer with whatever came first to mind.

The major focus of needs in South County was on medical services for the elderly. The elderly population is growing rapidly, and providing services to this special population permeated the comments. Comments reflected a multifaceted problem. Further, many elderly residents find it difficult to pay for medical care. They moved with their spouses to the area to retire. Then one spouse either died or became ill, and the remaining spouse is strapped for resources. Finally, the need for assisting elderly people in their homes was cited: bathing, cooking, cleaning, diet and nutrition, and other needs.

Respondents commented on various aspects of the problem. First, "Access to medical care for the elderly is the most important. We have a hospital and good doctors, but we have trouble with actual transportation in getting there, and many of these people are too old and frail to use public transportation, and North County is one hour away. The biggest problem is providing health services for the elderly who are strapped. They are retired, and their children have moved away. We need a range of services, including counseling, education, nutrition, and daily living skills. Also, there is a need for transportation for shopping and medical appointments. The biggest changes are to a major retirement center. The number of seniors is bigger. As more come, the problems of aging will be even bigger. We have many retirees in this area. A lot of people just live on Social Security, and they have trouble making ends meet. They come down here to live, and one spouse either gets sick or dies. The biggest problem is taking care of senior citizens, with nutrition, bathing, cooking, or whatever they need."

Cost and access were another pressing problem seen in South County. Rural poverty is serious, and many can't afford, or won't pay for, health insurance. One said that "the biggest problem is ability to pay for the services provided. There is nothing for those who can't pay, especially for prescriptions. Doctors won't accept them if they can't pay up front. They don't qualify for anything out there. A lot of them are transients." A second agreed: "People have an inability to afford good healthcare. They don't place enough emphasis on prevention, but wait until something happens. A lot of people around here have seasonal low wages." A third respondent said: "We have a lot of people here who don't have [health insurance], and because of that they don't seek medical attention when they need it," or, as another put it, "Having access [to healthcare] locally and figuring out how to pay for it." A fourth respondent said, "I'm not sure, but the biggest problem is assistance to those who can't afford healthcare, dental care, counseling, etc. There isn't any transportation and you can't get there unless you have a car."

Other needs were noted as well. First, alcohol and drug abuse: "Alcohol and other drug abuse are the biggest problems [because] they result in a poor attitude at school and hinder performance." Next, mental health services: "[The biggest problem is] consistent and stable resources for mental health services for substance abuse and psychological counseling. It is a problem because of the number of high school dropouts and because of alcohol-related crimes." Third, lack of basic health information: "[We need] more information on what is available. There is a lack of confidence about what people can get." Fourth, heart disease and cancer: "Heart disease leads the pack; most deaths are from heart problems and cancer. The biggest thing on the west side is a growing retirement community, with cancer and aging." Fifth, local healthcare: "The biggest need is for a doctor or clinic close by or in our community so the elderly can go there for emergencies or for tests. Many people here are on fixed incomes and don't drive. There is a need for convenience and there is a lack of transportation. There is only one area hospital and, for a lot of folks, it is a long haul to get there. A lot of seniors have to travel for healthcare. If they had an attack they would be in danger of not getting there on time." Sixth, environmental issues: "The biggest problem is liquid waste treatment. The sewer system is not adequate for the growing population. Development is loading up the septic systems. The soils are not adequate to receive it."

The needs cited for East County reflect a more heterogeneous social situation. Many respondents echoed the concerns of those serving South County: the need for cancer care, better water quality, improved access to healthcare, affordable healthcare insurance, better information, and improved transportation. However, there was a greater need seen for improved health and welfare for children and for more practitioners and facilities, mainly because of the area's greater distance from existing healthcare providers and facilities.

First, representatives of East County agencies pinpointed children's health and well-being: "It is apparent from the appearance of the kids in schools that we are having difficulty caring for our children. One of the biggest problems lies in the poor healthcare given young children. They are not being taken for routine care, due to their parents' lack of money." Cancer was identified as another problem in East County: "A lot of people are having cancer. It seems like a lot of them are coming up with it." A third was access to healthcare: "East County has no hospital and providers are few. We have a good sized county of 20,000, six school districts, and youth of 15–17 years. Most are at the poverty level." And, "There are too many poor people who can't afford healthcare. East County is a poor county and there is a lot of underinsurance." An agency rep said, "There is a lack of security over health insurance at the local level. Businesses try to budget for employees but have trouble doing so because of having to contract with insurance companies." Another said, "There is a lack of employers providing health insurance because of the cost of providing it, and the difficulty of people paying for it."

Finally, a group of miscellaneous needs. One was a need for more doctors: "There is a need for more physicians, particularly family practitioners. We have specialists near but not here." A second was water quality: "We have leaky infiltration systems—the most important problem. Too many old septic tanks are leaking into the lake." Third noted was, "There is a lack of information about family services and qualifying for Medicaid. People don't know how to place a relative because there aren't any straight answers." Finally: "We have transportation problems in getting to a doctor or a dentist from the outlying areas. There is transportation, as long as you don't count on getting where you want when you want it."

East County needs parallel North County as well: improved transportation, improved sex education, mental health services, more doctors, better prenatal care, and improved care for cancer and heart problems. With regard to transportation, one commented that "our major difficulty is transportation to get people to medical care. There aren't a lot of providers in our county, and getting to South County Hospital is difficult." Another saw as most pressing a "lack of sex education; there are lots of teens pregnant, but not much sexually transmitted diseases. Education is needed, but it is seen as a no, so it's difficult." A fourth noted: "Mental health services are needed. We have North County Mental Health Counseling Center, but staff is very limited. We tried to get a tax levy to support it, but it failed. We have a lot of abuse cases. And alcohol and drug dependency that falls to law enforcement and jail time should really be treated at the health center. There are no emergency services on off hours, and 45 minutes away." Fifth, more doctors: according to one respondent, "We need more doctors here in the immediate area. We have a new doctor coming in October. Now we need a GP." Another said, "We have a lack of doctors here after hours and on weekends. There are two clinics in town. In an emergency, we have to go 40 plus miles to a hospital. " A sixth reported a lack of prenatal care as the biggest problem: "A lot of people are on welfare, and don't get the help they need." Finally, cancer and heart care were most greatly needed: "We are losing a lot of people to cancer, and we have a lot of people with a heart condition."

Most interesting in this area was a need not identified as important: teenage pregnancy. No community leader in any of the three counties identified teenage pregnancy as a pressing health need. When leaders were asked about the importance of teenage pregnancy, some said that, while it was a very important problem, it was not of utmost importance. Others said it was not important at all. Here is a representative listing: "It isn't very important on my spectrum of problems"; "We have some of it, but not so bad as in the city"; "It is not very serious because of the type of population we have"; "I don't think we have a big problem with it"; "It is an important problem and getting worse, but it isn't at the top of the list"; "Teenage pregnancy is prevalent, but it's not that big a deal"; "Teenage pregnancy might rate a 7 or 8 on a 10-point scale"; "It rates about a 3 on a 1–10 scale [where 10 is highest]"; "on a 1–10 scale, I'd give it a 7 or 8"; "It is a problem, but not a serious one"; "It is definitely a problem, but probably not any worse than anywhere else"; "It is not a major problem, but somewhat of a problem"; and, "I think there is a lot of teenage pregnancy, and we have latch-key children, but I don't know that it is a big problem."

Next, we asked respondents to evaluate current efforts to meet or address the problems they had identified. Respondents quite candidly offered their evaluations of current efforts. In South County, interviewees gave a mixed review to efforts to meet the needs of the elderly. One was critical of current efforts: "Nothing is being done. Government has to look at it [the issue of inability to pay for services] more broadly, at expanding services for the elderly." Another agreed, saying: "Nothing is being done." Others reacted more favorably: "Meals on Wheels visits the elderly on a daily basis and offers frozen meals once a week. They assess their needs during the visit. It is doing pretty well by meeting the needs of 60 percent of the elderly." Another referred to several private home health agencies and county health departments that make available services for low-income elderly. "To my knowledge," he said, "they are doing a very adequate job, but there's always room for improvement." Another respondent agreed that the home health agencies do a good job. "They go in there to help them [the elderly] take care of themselves. People's opinions of them are good, as is the testimony of clients who have been served." One political leader thought that the efforts of South County Hospital are "moderately effective," because they can treat most illnesses. "Of course," he added, "in a lot of serious cases they make the decision to get them out of there." Another said that efforts to treat the elderly are adequate now, but that, when the physician on the west side of the lake retires, there will a problem in his part of the county.

With regard to meeting problems of transport in South County, respondents thought there seems to be little being done to improve the transportation system within the county so the elderly can get to medical and dental appointments: "We've been trying to get people to do it. The county passed the property tax funding transportation this year." Funds were limited, though. A popular solution posed is building more facilities in the outlying areas. "I have heard of clinics coming in," said one respondent, "some kind of doc in the shop kind of thing." According to another, "We've talked about it [getting a facility], and applied for a facility here, but we can't get one."

In helping increase people's ability to pay for health insurance or healthcare, respondents see very little being done in this area. "There's not much being done," said one. "The hospital is working on programs to develop a wellness attitude," said another, "but there is nothing organized." "The legislature is looking at costs and the best way to meet them," added another, "and the division of health is providing programs and services even though people don't have the money." "I can't say locally," said one respondent; "we as an employer are making every effort to provide insurance to our employees."

To meet the other needs, here are the actions cited by South County respondents, together with their evaluation of their adequacy. To address the need for more information about healthcare: "Nothing is being done." To improve the treatment of cancer: "Nothing is really happening. I'm sure there's lots of research, but I'm not aware of anything specific that's being done." To meet the need to combat alcohol and drug abuse: "In-school [antialcohol and other drug abuse] programs, such as DARE, Red Ribbon Week, and the School and Community Drug Team, are happening. It is always hard to know exactly how many people you've saved from going off the deep end." To beef up mental health services: "Resources are out there, but they don't cover a broad range, and they only concentrate on offending males and are short lived." To improve the area's sewer systems and liquid waste problems: "We're putting in sewer systems. Where they are in, they are adequate, but they are not being put in fast enough. But nothing is being done in the outlying areas to solve liquid waste problems. In the city we are working on grants to upgrade the system."

Respondents noted the following actions being taken to address health needs in East County. First, the East County Health Department provides a range of services for children. One respondent added, "They may be doing the most they can." Another respondent indicated that, "The health department is giving a grant to provide school health services to schools that don't have the funds." To alleviate the high cost of insurance and the lack of access to affordable health insurance, one respondent noted, "East County is looking at county insurance," but reflected a sense of futility: "A lot of people have looked at it, but can't afford to offer it." Another respondent noted that business organizations are making an effort to take the needs of small business to Congress, and that "NFIB is doing a good job." Still another pointed to "hospitals joining to get together to try to cut down costs by specializing," and placed the effort at "about 50 percent effective."

Other actions noted by respondents in East County are the following. To help with transportation: "The bus company runs." To increase the number of physicians: "A local clinic has attracted a young physician." To increase information about family services and qualifying for Medicaid: "Nothing is being done. There is an effort to hire someone with social services background to help with information." To stop the leaking of old septic systems into the lake: "We're trying to put them on the sewer system as much as we can. This is difficult due to the hilly nature of the area."

To address the need for more physicians in North County, the community is attempting to recruit physicians. "St. Mary's is working on it. There's only one general clinic. They're trying, but it isn't done yet." According to another: "There have been a number of meetings with Memorial Hospital. It seems that we can't pay enough for a doctor. To date, zero has come of it." To alleviate the dearth of transportation: "Nothing is being done. The bus is available to anyone on a sliding scale, but it doesn't go everywhere every day, and scheduling is difficult." To address the need for more mental health services: "The center is doing the best it can, but that's not adequate. It needs more money and more staff, especially as the case load increases."

By way of increasing teenagers' understanding of issues related to pregnancy: "There are efforts to cooperate with the schools, by sending nurses out, but I don't know where that stands." For cancer and heart care: "We've been having a doctor out of another county. I don't know about South County Hospital. It would be a big asset to have a hospital on each side of the lake. Our efforts are as adequate as they can get." To improve prenatal care in the county, one respondent pointed to a group of concerned citizens. "A levy has been shot down," he said. "They've gotten some private funds out there, but the levies have been voted down the last two times. The people could have helped themselves."

Next, we asked respondents to name the organization or agency that would be best equipped to meet these needs or to address the community health issues. There was a view taken by many respondents that the hospital should be involved in addressing the health status of the community, but there was no strong consensus in any of the counties we studied. In South County, six respondents said they did not know which agency or organization would be most appropriate for this task. Four specifically named the hospital in combination with other community organizations, because the hospital was seen as central to community effort: "the hospital because it is the focal point"; "the hospital, physicians, individuals, and the community itself," "a joint effort with ambulance services, doctors, and the hospital"; and "an organization in the loop that would be the hospital or tied to it." Other representatives identified the following organizations or agencies as most appropriate: the federal government, specialty physicians, home health agency and county health department, the court system, the chamber of commerce, county government, Citizens for Progress, the state and civic organizations, taxpayers, American Heart Association, the schools, and the county.

There was no consensus among East and North, either. In East County, two people did not know. Two individuals mentioned the health department, and one gave the hospital. Other organizations mentioned were: the city government, a variety of organizations (including the ministerial alliance), the county, OATS bus, county health department, the Division of Family Services, the health department and the school system, insurance companies and the hospital, NFIB and the Missouri Municipal League, and "the government." In North County, no one organization was favored. A hospital or clinic was mentioned by one person. Others included: the city and Memorial Hospital; "whoever has money"; government; parents, teachers, and children; county commissioners; and the state Mental Health Department. Three leaders said they didn't know.

We then asked respondents the following question: "How well would you say that South County Hospital is meeting the overall health needs or addressing these issues in this area? If you were to give them a grade, either A, B, C, D, or F, like in school, where an A is excellent and an F is failing, what would it be?"

Overall, South County Hospital was seen as doing an excellent job of meeting the health needs of the community. Where criticized, it was only because it was too far away or because it wasn't large enough.

In South County, South County Hospital received a grade point average of 3.14, about a B/B+, with 21 respondents grading, and one respondent refusing to offer a guess. Ten gave the hospital an A; 12 gave the hospital a B; and 7 gave the hospital a C. Below are displayed the open-ended comments of respondents:

> A lifesaver. One of the greatest things that ever happened to our community. They do a great job. People know it and believe in it. It has expanded its capabilities rather than being a satellite.

A terrific job. A few friends have been in the hospital. He's alive because it is well-equipped and expanding. I believe it is one of the best in the area.

It is doing a real good job, better for South County. People in North County prefer Jefferson. They have expanded their services, education department, and health fairs.

Excellent: I have seen them treat people and know the people who work there.

A marvelous hospital. They are doing everything they can with what they have. It is a top-rated hospital. They even keep the rates evened out. I have never found a doctor I haven't felt great about.

A very good job. They realize additional needs there. They try to position themselves so they can reach other people.

They do very well through educational programs. Also, excellent from a vocational perspective with health fairs.

They do very well. There is a lack of confidence on the part of the community in the facility, but it is a wonderful place. There isn't any public awareness of what goes on inside the place, though.

A good job. They are expanding to meet a growing population and have needed to upgrade staff to provide staff in other areas. In all of the areas, other than just the emergency room, they try to do an excellent job.

It does real well, providing a full line of services in most areas. Emergency room services can handle most everyday problems. A lot of more serious patients are sent to other hospitals. I don't know how well they can treat them.

They do a good job of education, care, and discharge planning for people who come into their facility. Most of those are from South County. They do some outreach in South County, but people in North County go to Sedalia or Jefferson City.

I haven't needed it as a patient, but it is getting more specialized care, more outpatient care. To get an A, they need to talk to the community about what they are doing.

They are doing a fairly good job. I've not had to use their services; but, if you have something that is moderately severe, you can go up to South County Hospital. It is difficult to get to the hospital. I don't know if it can get an A.

It's very good. The service is adequate. The facility is modern. They are upgrading it, adding services. It has its limitations. To get more than a B it would have to offer more services so that people don't have to be ferried away.

It's the only hospital there. Most feel it has come a long way and is improved. To get an A, it would have to get a higher degree of personnel competent in critical areas—radiology, oncology.

It is doing fairly well. There are so many agencies to work with. There are a lot of medical problems. A lot of people go to Columbia because there are not enough specialists. [To get an A] I think that everything should be done in the county.

I don't know. I don't get a lot of input. A lot of people go there for emergency situations. Not too many of the local people stay there, due to cost. The equipment is wonderful, but charges are the biggest problem. Cost comparison shows it to be very expensive.

It provides a facility people can come to which is doing an excellent job. It is criticized on cost. A lot of people go elsewhere. It has a problem with cost and not enough help, which makes it less desirable.

It is doing a fair job. There is a good variety of services to address that it couldn't do previously. In order to get an A, it needs to be more cost-efficient and do more outreach. Education effort to make more programs available at convenient times of day and days of week.

It is doing fairly well. The only thing I deal with is their emergency room. There is some improvement there, but they should be more respectful of the need for information and they should let escorts go in with patients to help them in the treatment rooms.

It is fair. It should offer more advanced technology and more doctors. They send them off to Jefferson City or to Columbia.

East County respondents gave much lower grades to the hospital: about a C+/B–, with five Bs, two Cs, and one D, primarily because the hospital was farther away. Respondents gave a variety of comments: (1) "It is doing a superior job. It is a nice facility, and is continually upgraded. There is a large specialty group there. It is too far away to get an A, simply because of traffic. They have a physician so it helps short of a satellite." (2) "We refer anyone who is looking for prenatal care to the hospital because it is closest. Our church refers people to the hospital in Columbia because it is cheaper. It is a good hospital, but it costs a lot to go there." (3) "It ought to do more outreach. If they are doing these things, I am not aware of it, and I usually know about these things." (4) "They do a good job on ER and trauma situations. Extended healthcare is not well-equipped for long-term hospitalizations. They do a good job for a small rural hospital. To get more than a B, they would have to do more long-term care." (5) "They do generally well. They offer free screening clinics and promote them appropriately. To do better than a B, they need to provide additional facilities to children's programs, additional wellness for children programs." (6) "I'm not that familiar with it, but those whom I've talked to say it is fine. I can't give it a higher grade because of its size. It is too small to offer more than they do now." (7) "It is adequate. It serves our needs, good emergency room and skilled nursing, good heart and rehab."

North County leaders graded the hospital at 2.71, about a C+, slightly higher than East County leaders, with five Bs and two Cs, primarily because the hospital is not as accessible as in South or North counties. Here are some quotes: (1) "The hospital needs to put more information out to us here on this side of the lake." (2) "In the southern part of the county it does a fantastic job, but not in the north. North City is closer and highways lead north more. Highway C is better than Route 54. Every hospital has its problems. I wouldn't give any hospital higher than a B." (3) "It's pretty good. Prenatal care folks prefer it. I have heard nothing but good things about it. It needs to reach out to the community. We need women's clinics there." (4) "It is doing a fine job. Some clientele will not go there. I don't know how many people go there. They tend to go to other hospitals because it is easier to get there. I wouldn't give them higher than a C because of a child abuse situation in which I couldn't get any information from them. I had to chase them down to get it." (5) "It is hard to judge. There is not much impact here; most people go to North City due to traffic. The health fairs are well received, but it could have more of a presence here through a satellite clinic. At most, a B–, unless they have a facility built here in Versailles." (6) "We are at the very south end of North County, and we aren't using them. Not higher than a C because of the attitude of the nurses. They do what they want, when they want to do it, not when it needs to be done. I'm basing my evaluation on just one incident." (7) "There are no facilities here. They offer nothing to us. Not higher than a C, until they have a satellite clinic that offers services that others don't."

Future Needs

To gain respondents' guesses of future needs, we asked community leaders: "Next, let's think about the county's needs 5 or 10 years down the road. What would you say will be the most pressing health problem at that point?" South County respondents identified three: care of the elderly, continued problems with access and cost, and long-term chronic illnesses.

A strong consensus held that care for the elderly in South County will be the most pressing need down the road. "We have a lot of couples coming here. Then one dies, or health fails, and there are problems," said one respondent. Another noted: "Old folks will put more pressure on the hospital, which will need more beds." And a third: "The hospital will have to enlarge its services. Taking care of the elderly will be the most important task; the sheer numbers will be crunching."

Related to increased need for care of the elderly will be a greater need for homecare—"keeping people independent at home." Additional geriatric specialists, more facilities, expanded hospital services, and other resources, education, counseling, and in-home assistance are all suggested by community leaders. Beyond this, the components of the medical delivery system will have to work more effectively with one another. In the words of one leader, "Better coordination for case management throughout the system will be needed. Right now, the system is very fragmented. Communication will have to be enhanced to have broader coverage. More services will have to be directed to the elderly to close the gaps."

Several leaders felt that the major issue to be addressed in the future will still be access and cost. The area will still have a large number of underinsured, and the area will need additional resources and facilities to increase access to medical services. In addition, there will have to be more public education, and more stress on preventive care as well as more money for treatment.

AIDS and other sexually transmitted diseases, along with Alzheimer and dementia, will be pressing issues in the future. Education and more outreach clinics in smaller areas will be needed to deal with these more difficult conditions. Above all, more resources will have to be devoted to addressing each of these problems.

In East County the need for affordable healthcare is seen as the most pressing future need. "There will still be a need for preventive healthcare for those who can afford to do it—taking kids in for shots, etc." Another added, "We will still have people who need healthcare. The problem will be the same, and possibly worse." There was a strong sentiment that any solution to this problem was out of the hands of people in the county. "Political decisions will rest at the executive level in Washington," said one. Public education to raise awareness around the issue together with economic assistance would be important. Other future problems noted include the following: (1) "AIDS, probably, will be a big one. We need education to deal with it." (2) "Cancer and heart will be the major ones. To address it, we will need a change in behavior—more exercise, better diet. I don't know, you can warn people a hundred times, but they don't do anything. Education would be important." (3) "Adult daycare services and additional residential care will be major needs. We need to get money from Medicare/Medicaid. The answer also lies in government reform." (4) "Children and elderly wellness will be big problems. We'll see an influx of retirees. We'll have to have some aid from the state as well as be able to handle increased volume at the hospital and clinics." (5) "We'll need a strong law enforcement commitment to exert more resources. That will take money." (6) "Drug and substance abuse as well as a proliferation of teen pregnancies, etc. Education is the answer to a lot of the problems, educational programs and prevention programs. We need to start young and fire point blank."

Community leaders in North County stressed the need for geriatric services: "The growth rate [among the elderly] is going to be real high. We're becoming a retirement center." "The projections are for more elderly and for less youth," noted another. And a third pointed to a growth in year-rounders, particularly those seeking geriatric services: "Folks will need a clinic branch of the hospital." Most community leaders saw increased hospital services and the building of satellite clinics as an answer, as well as increased homecare services so people don't have to enter a nursing home.

Other needs mentioned for North County were: (1) "Teen pregnancy will multiply and be really big; also HIV and tuberculosis. We'll need education and increased emphasis on prevention." (2) "Transportation, if nothing happens. We'll need some kind of countywide system to connect people to other medical facilities." (3) "There will be a need for more GPs. We're close to Columbia for specialists." (4) "Mental health issues will be the key. We will need to build a full facility here that includes a range of mental health services as well as traditional services."

To gain further understanding of how community leaders feel about the hospital, we asked them about how well the local hospital was planning to provide for meeting people's needs in the future. South County respondents responded largely in a positive vein: (1) "They're doing good. They have a lot of programs to help people with diabetes or whatever they need." (2) "There are constantly new things coming." (3) "With the building program and what's been added in the past year or two, a new wing and outpatient services. They're bringing in specialists and establishing a skilled nursing facility." (4) "They're doing well to expand as needs grow.

They are trying to build a facility which will be up to meeting the needs in the future." (5) "From what I've heard, they are very focused and visionary, building new additions and so forth." (6) "They have added to the hospital and greatly expanded it, and they also do outreach to the community, wellness, etc." (7) "I can't say enough about their progress and improvements because I know where they are coming from." (8) "They will be well equipped to meet anything. They have good doctors, etc. It will continue to be one of the best facilities." (9) "They are at the top of the list in that area, adding new facilities, equipment, etc."

East County respondents, farther away from the hospital, have had fewer dealings with it and had less of a sense of the hospital's planning efforts. One said, "I don't know"; another said: "I am not familiar [enough] with them to know what they are doing." Of the three that expressed an opinion, one thought they were doing well by adding more doctors and specialists; another said the hospital is doing "as well as or better than any provider in the area with expanded newborn and other programs"; and a third said that he thought it was doing reasonably well, but that "I'm not that familiar with it. I'm going on what I hear in conversation, and no one is ecstatic about it either way."

Only one representative in East County expressed an opinion: "They are doing quite well with an active volunteer organization, a community-minded board that gets out often to promote the hospital."

To conclude the interview, we asked respondents, "If I were the CEO of South County Hospital and asked you for advice, what is the most important advice you could give me?" Community organizations and leaders clearly want a community hospital that will work with them in partnership for the community. Some of their responses were: (1) "Keep up the good work. Stay people-oriented." (2) "Communicate with each element of the healthcare delivery system so they can work together most effectively." (3) "Keep from succumbing to tunnel vision and not really seeing the big picture." (4) "Do more public education and try to get out and work more closely with agencies in the community."

Many East County respondents said the same thing: (1) "Be in touch with the public, in every realm you work with." (2) "Do better public relations, and have more outreach to community." (3) "I want to see networking with the hospital so we could work together to provide services for the community. Too often we're in competition when we shouldn't be."

East County respondents want the hospital to pay more attention to them: (1) "Keep attention to all areas of the lake. Broaden it more into

North County, more than they are now. Run a good campaign, and promote better to highlight the hospital's different services." (2) "Come here on clinic days. I would like to sit down and talk with you to see what we could do together." (3) "Build a satellite clinic that will take care of the needs in this county."

HEALTH PATTERNS AND PRACTICES IN THE ASSESSMENT AREA

The third section of this chapter presents the results of a telephone survey of households in South, East, and North counties conducted during the summer of 1994. Those interviewed were involved in making decisions for their households. Random numbers were supplied by a firm that specializes in providing random number samples to market research companies and other organizations doing market research. Interviews were conducted in proportion to households contributed by each county to the total number of households in the survey area. For samples of this size, a maximum expected statistical error, for the three-county area, is +/– 5.0 percentage points at the 95 percent confidence level. This means that, if the study were replicated "N" times, the results for each item would be within 5.0 percentage points, high or low, of the observed result in 95 times out of 100 replications. The maximum expected statistical error is +/– 9.5 percentage points for South County, +/- 10 percentage points for East County, and +/– 10.0 percentage points for North County.

Sampling is always vulnerable to statistical error. Therefore, the reader should be careful when interpreting these findings. They are accurate, but precise only within the stated margins of error. One should interpret these results carefully and guard against attributing excess concreteness to differences among small subgroups. These subgroups may have larger margins of error associated with them.

Households and Respondents Compared

Exhibit 2–2 displays the population of the assessment area by total and county, and the number of completed interviews by total and by county, together with the sample variation. Results show that South County is almost precisely represented, East County is slightly underrepresented, and North County is slightly under overrepresented. Sample variation is not statistically significant.

EXHIBIT 2–2
Total Households and Survey Respondents

County	Percent of Households	Percent of Interviews	Difference
South	44.2%	41.1%	3.1%
East	31.2	30.3	0.9
North	24.6	28.6	(4.0)
Total	100.0	100.0	0.0

Characteristics of Respondents

This section shows the breakdown on selected demographic variables from the community survey. The results are reliable for the three counties as a whole, within a margin of error of 5.0 percentage points, high or low. Unless noted otherwise, there were no substantial or statistically significant variations by county.

Employment

About 6.1 percent of survey respondents report being unemployed. This approximates the percentage of respondents given as unemployed by the census, though there were some variations. Survey results are consistent with census data to the extent that proportionately fewer South County residents report being out of work. About 31.9 percent of survey respondents report an age of over 65, and 11.6 percent report being over 75. These data reflect a significantly higher proportion of respondents over the age of 65 years than we would have expected by examining the 1990 census data. According to census data presented in Exhibit 2–3, 17.5 percent of the area are aged 65 years or over, but the discrepancy probably can be explained by a high in-migration rate of retirement-age people, and an increased propensity of older residents to participate in surveys of all sorts.

Despite the recent growing in-migration of new residents, most respondents are long-term residents. Almost 40 percent have lived in the area for 20 or more years; 60.7 percent have lived there for 10 or more years. About 2.9 percent have lived in the area over less than one year.

EXHIBIT 2–3
Demographic Profile
Central Missouri, 1994

Characteristic

Number of years:

Less than 1 year	2.9
1 to 2 years	8.7
3 to 4 years	9.5
5 to 9 years	17.4
10 to 19 years	20.8
20 or more years	39.9
Refused	0.8

Age last birthday:

18 to 34	19.2
35 to 54	29.7
55 to 64	18.9
65 to 74	20.3
75 or over	11.6
Refused	0.3

Gender:

Male	32.6
Female	67.4

Employment:

Student	2.9
Outside home	36.6
In the home	6.6
Self-employed	7.6
Unemp. less than 1 yr.	2.4
Unemp. more than 1 yr.	3.7
Retired	39.9
Refused	0.3

Percent response

The Hospital's Share of Mind

The community hospital's share of mind is one measure of the health of a community. To measure the awareness of South County Hospital, we asked respondents: "Please name all the hospitals you can think of in your area." We recorded up to the first three hospitals mentioned. Reviewing the distribution of mentions across the hospitals selected suggests that respondents' definition of their area includes the major cities on the north and south. Looking at the percentage of first mentions shows South County Hospital with 57.1 percent of first mentions and 68.3 percent of all mentions. The next most frequently mentioned hospital was mentioned first by 8.3 percent of respondents and accounts for 40.7 percent of all mentions. These figures speak well for the hospital and show that the hospital is a focus of community attention. (See Exhibit 2–4.)

The Community's Evaluation of Its Community Hospital

Health status is enhanced when the community regards the hospital in a positive fashion. To measure the community's perception of the hospital, respondents were asked: "If you were to grade the hospital, like in school, what grade would you give it?" The hospital earned an overall grade of 3.39, slightly higher than a B+. Overall, the hospital was given a grade of about B/B+, 3.39 on a four-point grading scale, where 4 was an A and 0 was an F. About 19.5 percent gave the hospital an A, and 5.9 percent gave it less than an F. About 80.5 percent gave it less than an A; 22.3 percent indicated they did not know enough about the hospital to grade it. In North County the hospital achieved the highest grade point average, with an average grade of 3.76, or about A–; the hospital's grades were lowest among East County residents, at 3.12, or about a B/B+; South County residents gave the hospital a 3.39 grade point average. (See Exhibit 2-5.)

The Community's Services of Patients: Inpatient, Outpatient, Emergency Care

To understand the nature of past hospitalization experiences with health-care providers in the area, we asked a series of questions about people's hospitalization at area hospitals. Respondents were asked how long it had been since they used each kind of service. About 85.1 percent have used a hospital at some point in their lives, 19.4 percent within the past year, 29.9 percent within the past two years, and 41.8 percent within the past

EXHIBIT 2–4
Awareness of Hospitals
Central Missouri, 1994

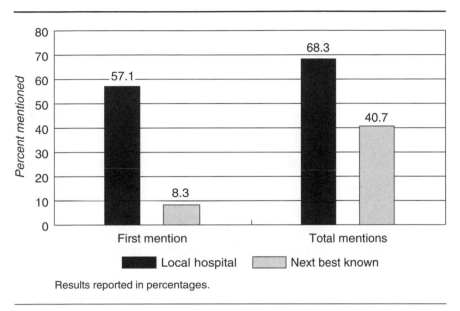

Results reported in percentages.

five years. About 15.6 percent have never used a hospital. About 31.3 percent have never used a hospital's outpatient services. About 68.7 percent
have used outpatient services sometime in the past, 53.7 within the past
five years, 44.0 percent within the past two years, and 33.3 percent within
the past year. About 2.5 percent say they have used outpatient services,
but they do not remember when. About 62.9 percent have used a hospital's emergency room. Almost 42 percent have done so within the past five
years, 29.6 percent within the past two years, and 20.1 percent during the
past year. About 2.0 percent have used an emergency room but do not
remember when. About 37.1 percent have never used an emergency room.
(See Exhibit 2–6.)

The Share of Patients of the Community's Hospital

Use of the local hospital is another indicator of community health. Where
the community hospital provides a focus for the community, where it is well
regarded, and where people use the local hospital, the health environment is

EXHIBIT 2–5
Grades for Local Hospital
Central Missouri, 1994

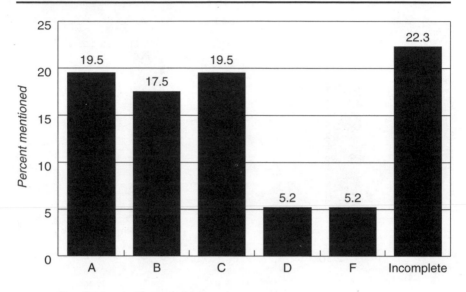

Results reported in percentages.
Based on respondents mentioning Central Missouri Hospital.

enhanced. Therefore, we asked those respondents who had used a hospital which hospital they had used for each kind of service. South County Hospital's share of patients was highest in each category, though lowest for inpatient care. For inpatient services, South County Hospital headed the list of area hospitals used, with 15.5 percent of all mentions. The next most often used hospital accounted for 11.4 percent of respondents. Next, for outpatient services, 27.2 percent of respondents have used South County Hospital; 11.6 have used the next most often used hospital. Finally, 34.4 percent of all respondents had used the emergency room of South County Hospital; only 7.5 percent had used the next most used hospital.

Health Status Indicator: Satisfaction with Services

A final indicator related to hospital use is the satisfaction with services received. Where people are satisfied with the services of their community hospital, the status of the community is enhanced. To measure the public's

EXHIBIT 2–6
Use of Inpatient, Outpatient, and ER Care
Central Missouri, 1994

Service used

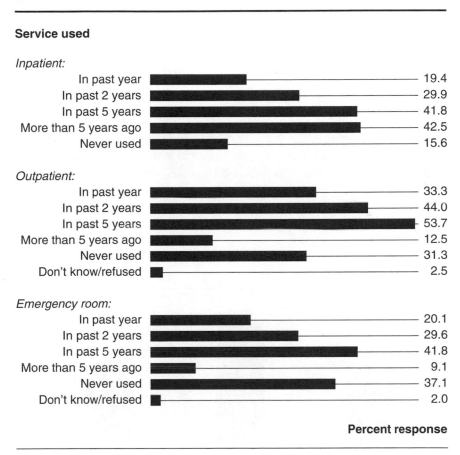

Inpatient:
In past year	19.4
In past 2 years	29.9
In past 5 years	41.8
More than 5 years ago	42.5
Never used	15.6

Outpatient:
In past year	33.3
In past 2 years	44.0
In past 5 years	53.7
More than 5 years ago	12.5
Never used	31.3
Don't know/refused	2.5

Emergency room:
In past year	20.1
In past 2 years	29.6
In past 5 years	41.8
More than 5 years ago	9.1
Never used	37.1
Don't know/refused	2.0

Percent response

satisfaction with services they had received, we asked those who had used each hospital for inpatient care to indicate how likely they might be to return to that hospital for hospitalization. Adding, for each hospital used, the percentage of people who indicated they would be very likely to return to the percentage who indicated they would be somewhat likely to return gave a kind of patient satisfaction score, the highest value of which equals 100.

Satisfaction scores for all hospitals used were quite low in the area studied. Looking at the percentage of people who report being very or somewhat likely to return for all hospitals used shows a satisfaction level of 59.0 percent for inpatient services, 72.0 for outpatient services, and 58.7 for emergency rooms visited. Comparable figures for Central County Hospital were 63.5 percent for inpatient services, 74.0 for outpatient services, and 58.0 for emergency room. That is, South County Hospital was rated about the same as all other hospitals for inpatient and emergency room services, and slightly better than other hospitals for outpatient services. (See Exhibit 2–7.)

Pressing Health Problems in the Community

To gather community input regarding key healthcare concerns, we asked respondents to tell us what they felt were the most pressing health concerns in their community. About 24.1 percent said they don't know. Of the rest, 13.9 gave heart problems, 13.9 percent said cancer care, and 6.9 per-

EXHIBIT 2–7
Satisfaction with Care
Central Missouri, 1994

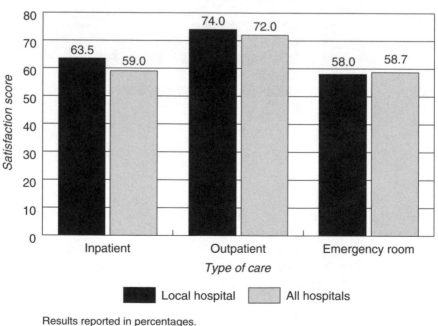

Results reported in percentages.

cent cited problems related to the elderly. About 4.9 percent thought the area had no health problems. (See Exhibit 2–8.)

Medical Services Needed Most in the Community

As a followup, we asked study participants to indicate the medical services they thought would be needed more in the community. Again, about one-quarter gave a "don't know" response. About 18.9 percent cited the need for more doctors, 5.2 percent wanted more services or better care for the elderly, and 4.2 percent wanted closer doctors or specialists. About 2 percent thought the area needed "everything," and 11.7 percent thought no additional services were needed in the area. Exhibit 2–9 gives these data as well as a comprehensive list of other services noted.

EXHIBIT 2–8
Perception of Key Health Needs
Central Missouri, 1994

Perceived need

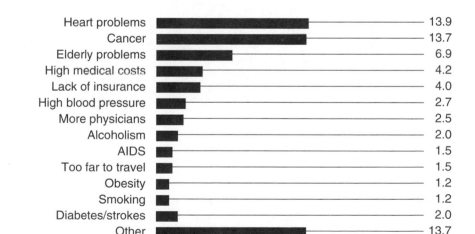

Heart problems	13.9
Cancer	13.7
Elderly problems	6.9
High medical costs	4.2
Lack of insurance	4.0
High blood pressure	2.7
More physicians	2.5
Alcoholism	2.0
AIDS	1.5
Too far to travel	1.5
Obesity	1.2
Smoking	1.2
Diabetes/strokes	2.0
Other	13.7
Don't know	24.1
None	4.9

Percent response

EXHIBIT 2–9
Perception of Needed Services
Central Missouri, 1994

Service needed

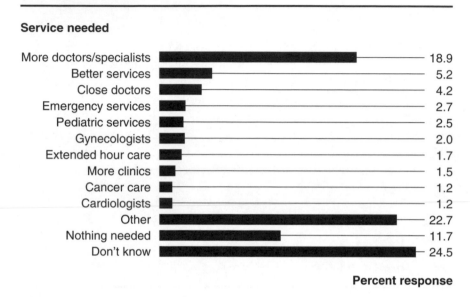

More doctors/specialists	18.9
Better services	5.2
Close doctors	4.2
Emergency services	2.7
Pediatric services	2.5
Gynecologists	2.0
Extended hour care	1.7
More clinics	1.5
Cancer care	1.2
Cardiologists	1.2
Other	22.7
Nothing needed	11.7
Don't know	24.5

Percent response

Delaying Doctors' Visits

About 9 percent report having delayed visiting a doctor because of cost.

Overview of Health-Related Behavior

The remaining section of this chapter presents the results from a series of questions probing the incidence of specific behaviors often referred to as health status indicators. A survey of these behaviors pinpoints the existence of behaviors which, if changed, could markedly improve the health status of the community and make it a healthier and better place to live. Questions were selected from the behavior risk surveillance questionnaire administered nationwide through the various state departments of health. Results for South, East, and North counties have been compared with statewide data in Exhibit 2–22.

Data from our study have been compared with state and national data, where warranted. In some cases, data were not available, and in others differences in the wording of questions made comparisons problematic. Statewide data have been taken from the statewide behavioral risk survey conducted through the Missouri Department of Health, and national data have been taken from studies quoted in *Healthy People 2000*.[1] Whenever possible, we have quoted specific studies from *Healthy People 2000*; but where specific studies are not referenced, we have referred to the appropriate page in the document itself. In Exhibit 2–22 (page 61), I have summarized all those variables on which those variations are statistically significant.

Safety Belt Usage

National research has shown that using safety belts has a dramatic effect on increasing life expectancy in a community. National health promotion and disease prevention objectives, hereafter referred to as national objectives, have set as a goal that, by the year 2000, 95 percent of all riders or drivers should be using seat belts.[2] Our results show that about 65.9 percent of respondents "always" use their seat belts when they drive a car or ride in a car. Another 15.7 percent report nearly always wearing seat belts; 7.2 percent sometimes do so; 5.7 say they rarely use one; and about 5.0 percent say they never wear their seat belt. Safety belt usage in the assessment area is significantly below the state average. (See Exhibit 2–10.)

EXHIBIT 2–10
Seat Belt Usage
Central Missouri, 1994

Wear belt...

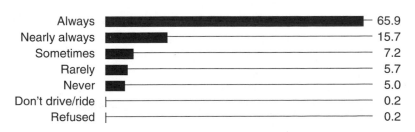

	Percent response
Always	65.9
Nearly always	15.7
Sometimes	7.2
Rarely	5.7
Never	5.0
Don't drive/ride	0.2
Refused	0.2

Blood Pressure

It is known that long-term blood pressure control can help to reduce the incidence of and death caused by cardiovascular diseases, such as coronary heart disease, hypertensive heart disease, and stroke. National research shows blood pressure control is improving to the point that the Long-Range Planning Committee of the National High Blood Pressure Education Program has set as a goal for the year 2000 that 50 percent of people should have their blood pressure "under control."[3] Our results are not conclusive in this matter, because we do not know how many people have had their blood pressure checked. However, blood pressure checks are routine in most physicals. Almost everyone in the area has visited a doctor at some time in their lives, so it may be safe to conclude that the proportion of people who have been diagnosed with high blood pressure is well below the goal of 50 percent. Exhibit 2–11 further shows us that almost three-quarters of those with high blood pressure are taking some form of medication to control it. The proportion of people reporting they have never been told they have high blood pressure is higher than the state average, but not significantly.

Exercise

By now significant evidence points to the many health benefits of regular physical activity. Exercise and physical activity can help to control coronary heart disease, hypertension, noninsulin-dependent diabetes, osteoporosis, obesity, and depression. Some studies have linked greater physical activity with lower rates of stroke, colon cancer, and reduced back injuries. Further, increasing evidence shows that even low to moderate exercise can have significant health benefits.[4] We asked respondents: "On what type of physical activity did you spend the most time during the past month." About 69.6 percent engaged in some form of activity. Of those engaging in activities, 64.0 percent named walking; 5.9 percent cited running or jogging; 4.8 percent named golf; 3.5 percent gave bicycling and physical training. Less commonly mentioned were swimming, using home exercisers, aerobics, softball, and gardening. To gain an overall measure of the level of physical activity in the study area, we asked respondents about how many times per week or per month each participated in the activity. We then asked about how many hours or minutes they kept at it when they took part in the activity. Looking at the sample

EXHIBIT 2–11
High Blood Pressure
Central Missouri, 1994

Question

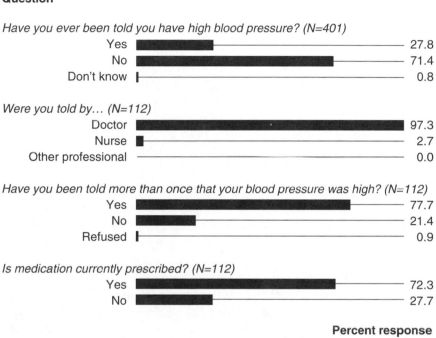

Have you ever been told you have high blood pressure? (N=401)

Yes	27.8
No	71.4
Don't know	0.8

Were you told by... (N=112)

Doctor	97.3
Nurse	2.7
Other professional	0.0

Have you been told more than once that your blood pressure was high? (N=112)

Yes	77.7
No	21.4
Refused	0.9

Is medication currently prescribed? (N=112)

Yes	72.3
No	27.7

Percent response

as a whole, we found that respondents spent, on average, about 0.85 hours per session and exercised 2.9 times per week on average. As shown in Exhibit 2–12, this works out to an average of 2.45 hours per week of exercise per person. The proportion of survey respondents is higher than the statewide average, but not significantly.

Diet

Dietary factors contribute substantially to the incidence of preventable conditions and premature deaths in this country. Diet is linked to coronary heart disease, some types of cancer, strokes, noninsulin-dependent diabetes, and atherosclerosis. In addition, the Public Health Service has noted the disproportionate consumption of foods that are high in fat at the expense of consumption of healthier foods that are high in dietary fiber and high in complex carbohydrates.[5] Accordingly, a worthy objective for a population is to emphasize sound dietary practices combined with regular physical activity to attain an appropriate body weight.[6] The results of this study reveal that about 33.6 percent of respondents are trying to lose weight. About 32.6 percent of those who said they are attempting to control their weight are only attempting to consume fewer calories, about 5.2 percent are trying to increase their physical activity, and 46.7 percent are working on both approaches. Although our measures of diet control are not consistent with those outlined in *Healthy People 2000*, our results suggest that people are moving in the right direction. Data on diet are not available from the state. (See Exhibit 2–12.)

Smoking

Tobacco has been shown to be responsible for about one of six deaths in the United States and accounts for the single greatest source of preventable deaths.[7] The specific effects of smoking include low birth weight babies, up to 14 percent preterm deliveries, and about 10 percent of all infant deaths. The other effects of smoking have been documented in agonizing detail, and they therefore require little attention here. Over the past 25 years, total and per capita smoking has declined steadily from 40 percent in 1965 to 29 percent in 1987. Nevertheless, about one-third of adults continue to smoke, though that percentage is higher among men, blacks, blue-collar workers, and people with fewer years of education.[8] The county prevalence of smoking in the South–East–North area far exceeds the national average. About 50.7 percent of those who have smoked more than 100 cigarettes in their lives smoke now. About 61.5 percent started as a teenager, and about 45.8 percent smoke from 20 to 29 cigarettes per day. The proportion of smokers in the assessment is significantly higher than the state average. (See Exhibit 2–13.)

Alcohol Consumption

Research has shown that the impact made on our national health by alcohol has been "staggering." One 1983 study placed the costs of health problems related to alcohol at more than $70 billion. A study published in 1989 linked alcohol to nearly half of all deaths caused by motor vehicle

EXHIBIT 2–12
Diet and Exercise
Central Missouri, 1994

Question

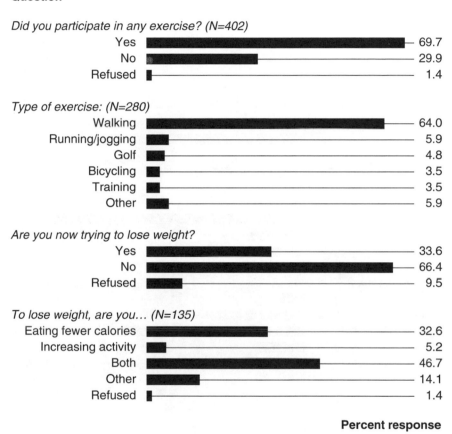

Did you participate in any exercise? (N=402)

Yes	69.7
No	29.9
Refused	1.4

Type of exercise: (N=280)

Walking	64.0
Running/jogging	5.9
Golf	4.8
Bicycling	3.5
Training	3.5
Other	5.9

Are you now trying to lose weight?

Yes	33.6
No	66.4
Refused	9.5

To lose weight, are you… (N=135)

Eating fewer calories	32.6
Increasing activity	5.2
Both	46.7
Other	14.1
Refused	1.4

Percent response

accidents and by fatal intentional injuries, such as suicides and homicides, drowning and boating deaths. Further, cirrhosis of the liver, largely attributable to heavy alcohol consumption, was the ninth leading cause of death in 1985. Adolescent users of alcohol and other drugs are more likely than nonusing teens to experience school failure, unwanted pregnancy, and delinquency. Abuse of alcohol significantly increases the risk of transmit-

EXHIBIT 2–13
Prevalence of Smoking
Central Missouri, 1994

Question

Have you smoked at least 100 cigarettes in your lifetime? (N=402)

Yes	55.5
No	44.0
Don't know	0.5

Do you smoke now? (N=223)

Yes	50.7
No	49.3

How old were you when you started to smoke regularly? (N=218)

Under 10	1.4
10 to 14	13.3
15 to 19	61.5
20 to 24	14.3
25 or over	9.5

Number of cigarettes smoked per day: (N=107)

1 to 9	7.5
10 to 19	24.3
20 to 29	45.8
30 to 39	12.1
More than 39	13.8

Percent response

---

ting the HIV virus through sharing contaminated needles, sexual contact with infected partners, or adverse affects of other unsafe sexual practices.[9]

Our results show that about 36.3 percent have had alcohol within the past month, on average about five occasions per month, with one to two drinks per occasion. Extrapolating from the data, the "average" person drinks about eight drinks per month. The proportion of people drinking five or more drinks on one occasion is significantly higher than the state average. (See Exhibit 2-14.)

EXHIBIT 2–14
Consumption of Alcohol
Central Missouri, 1994

Question

Have you had any alcohol in the past month? (N=402)

Yes — 36.3
No/don't know/refused — 63.7

How many days per month do you drink? (N=134)

Less than 5 — 46.3
5 to 9 — 29.1
More than 9 — 24.6

How many drinks per occasion do you have on average? (N=137)

1 — 34.3
2 — 29.2
3 — 16.8
More than 3 — 19.7

On how many occasions during the past mo. did you have more than 4? (N=137)

1 — 35.3
2 — 21.6
3-4 — 21.6
More than 4 — 22.5

Percent response

Physician Practices and Patterns

All but 1 percent have visited a physician at some time in their lives. About 81.3 percent visited a physician within the past year, 89.3 percent within the past two years, and 95.3 percent within the past five years. About 77.6 percent say they have a doctor they see regularly. About 13.6 percent of respondents indicated having had trouble finding a doctor. Of those who reported problems finding a physician, about 11.1 percent cited difficulties with finding a doctor who would take new patients, and 70.4 percent cited other reasons. About 15.8 percent had difficulty finding a specialist. Specialists most often sought were in gynecology and orthopedics. About 71.4 percent gave difficulties with transportation as the primary reason they couldn't find a specialist. (See Exhibit 2–15.)

EXHIBIT 2–15
Physician Patterns
Central Missouri, 1994

Question

How long since you last saw a doctor?

Ever	98.3
Within past 5 years	95.3
Within past 2 years	89.3
Within past year	81.3
Never	1.0
Don't know	0.7

Do you have a doctor you see regularly?

Yes	77.6
No	22.1
Don't know	0.3

Had trouble finding a general physician?

Yes	13.6
No	83.7
Don't know/refused	2.9

Had any trouble finding a specialist?

Yes	15.8
No	79.1
Don't know/refused	5.1

Percent response

Cholesterol

Over the past generation, the death rate due to cardiovascular disease has declined sharply, by more than 35 percent for all cardiovascular diseases, 40 percent for coronary heart disease, and 50 percent for strokes. High cholesterol is a major risk factor for cardiovascular disease, along with high blood pressure and smoking. Still, cardiovascular diseases kill as many people as all other diseases combined. Nationally, approximately 30 percent of adults have high cholesterol.[10] In the area studied here, about 78.3 percent of respondents have had their blood cholesterol checked sometime in their lives, 75.8 percent within the past five years, 67.6 percent within the past two years, and 57.2 percent within the past year. About 17.9 percent report never having had their blood cholesterol checked, and 3.7 percent have done so but can't remember when. Of those who have had their blood cholesterol checked, 71.4 percent have been told their level and 38.7 percent have been told their blood cholesterol level is too high. The proportion of people having had their cholesterol checked within the past five years is significantly higher than the state proportion. (See Exhibit 2–16.)

EXHIBIT 2–16
Blood Cholesterol
Central Missouri, 1994

Question

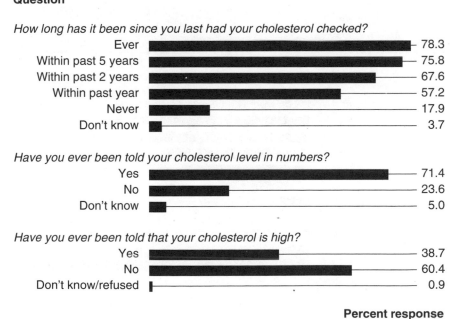

How long has it been since you last had your cholesterol checked?

	Percent
Ever	78.3
Within past 5 years	75.8
Within past 2 years	67.6
Within past year	57.2
Never	17.9
Don't know	3.7

Have you ever been told your cholesterol level in numbers?

	Percent
Yes	71.4
No	23.6
Don't know	5.0

Have you ever been told that your cholesterol is high?

	Percent
Yes	38.7
No	60.4
Don't know/refused	0.9

Percent response

Diabetes

About 7 million Americans suffer from diabetes. About 5 million more may have the disease without knowing it. Each year, about 650,000 new cases are discovered. Diabetes has been linked directly to over 37,000 deaths and indirectly to an additional 100,000. Diabetics face not only a shorter life but acute, chronic, and recurring complications. In 1987, patients with diabetes or related complications spent 9 million days in a hospital. The costs of diabetes were conservatively estimated at $20.4 billion in 1987.[11] The Public Health Service has given as a goal the reduction of the incidence of diabetes to no more than 25 persons per 1,000 people.[12] From our study, 29.9 percent of respondents have never been checked for diabetes. Of those who have been checked, 56.7 percent have been checked within the past five years, 49.5 percent within the past two years, 43.3 percent within the past year, and 10 percent have been checked but are not sure when. Of those who report having been checked, 11.6 percent were told that they have diabetes. This figure represents about 69.9 persons per thousand. The proportion of people diagnosed with diabetes is significantly higher than the statewide figure. (See Exhibit 2–17.)

EXHIBIT 2–17
Diabetes Screening
Central Missouri, 1994

Question

How long has it been since you were last checked for diabetes?

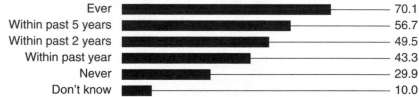

Ever	70.1
Within past 5 years	56.7
Within past 2 years	49.5
Within past year	43.3
Never	29.9
Don't know	10.0

Ever been told by a doctor or other healthcare worker you have diabetes?

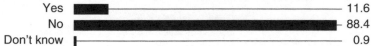

Yes	11.6
No	88.4
Don't know	0.9

Percent response

Health Insurance

About 77.4 percent of respondents report having some kind of healthcare insurance plan. Of those plans in force, 95.5 percent cover at least some hospital bills, 83.5 percent cover the cost of some doctor visits, and 72.9 percent cover some other expenses. The proportion of people without health insurance is significantly higher than statewide. (See Exhibit 2–18.)

Awareness of the HIV Virus and Related Issues

The HIV epidemic is a national crisis and international problem. Without treatment, within 10 years of infection, about 50 percent of the infected population will develop AIDS, and another 40 percent will develop other illnesses related to the HIV virus. In 1990, it was estimated that approximately 1 million Americans have been infected, at least 40,000 of them having become infected in 1989. HIV and AIDS constitute a growing and insidious threat to the fabric of society, and they will continue to make major demands on health and social systems for decades to come. Annual costs of AIDS are expected to exceed $13 billion, not including the costs of expanding the use of antiviral drugs, such as AZT.[13] (See Exhibit 2–19.)

Because of the seriousness of the problem, we felt it likely that AIDS may pose a threat to the medical service delivery system in the South City area. Before developing specific prevention and control strategies, it would be important to gain some understanding of the degree to which the public's understanding of the HIV epidemic is accurate. We first asked respondents: "Have you ever heard of the AIDS virus, also called by the name HIV?" Just over 96 percent said they had. We followed this question with a series of questions to measure the accuracy of the public's understanding of the problem: (1) "Do you think that a person who is infected with the AIDS virus can look and feel well and healthy?" (2) "Do you think a person can get infected with the AIDS virus from donating blood?" (3) "Do you think a person can get infected with the AIDS virus from being cared for by a healthcare worker who has the virus?" And (4) "How effective do you think using a condom is in preventing transmission of the AIDS virus through sexual activity?" About 77.5 percent think an infected person can look and feel healthy; 38.2 percent think a person can contract AIDS from donating blood; 58.1 percent think that a person can get AIDS from a healthcare worker; and 24.8 percent think that a condom is very effective in preventing one from con-

EXHIBIT 2–18
Health Insurance
Central Missouri, 1994

Question

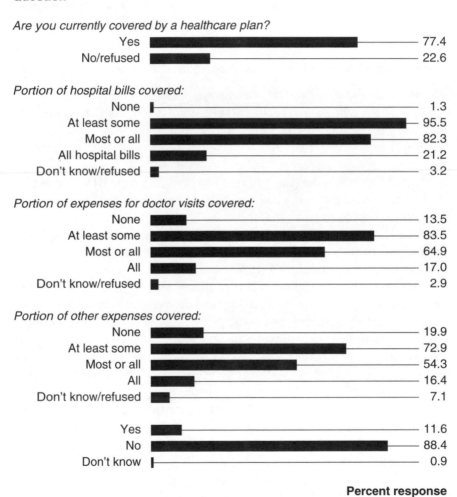

Are you currently covered by a healthcare plan?

Yes	77.4
No/refused	22.6

Portion of hospital bills covered:

None	1.3
At least some	95.5
Most or all	82.3
All hospital bills	21.2
Don't know/refused	3.2

Portion of expenses for doctor visits covered:

None	13.5
At least some	83.5
Most or all	64.9
All	17.0
Don't know/refused	2.9

Portion of other expenses covered:

None	19.9
At least some	72.9
Most or all	54.3
All	16.4
Don't know/refused	7.1

Yes	11.6
No	88.4
Don't know	0.9

Percent response

tracting AIDS. The proportion of people who say that a person with the HIV virus can look well and feel healthy is significantly higher than statewide data. The proportion of people who say that a condom is very

EXHIBIT 2–19
Awareness of HIV and Related Issues
Central Missouri, 1994

Question

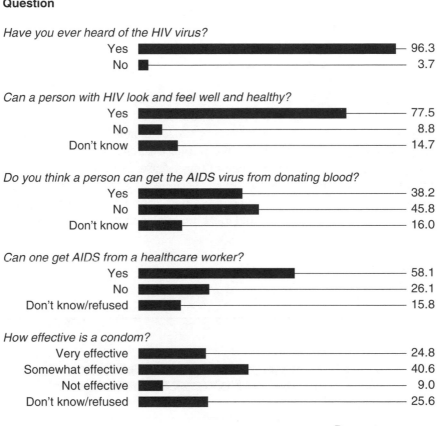

Have you ever heard of the HIV virus?

Yes — 96.3
No — 3.7

Can a person with HIV look and feel well and healthy?

Yes — 77.5
No — 8.8
Don't know — 14.7

Do you think a person can get the AIDS virus from donating blood?

Yes — 38.2
No — 45.8
Don't know — 16.0

Can one get AIDS from a healthcare worker?

Yes — 58.1
No — 26.1
Don't know/refused — 15.8

How effective is a condom?

Very effective — 24.8
Somewhat effective — 40.6
Not effective — 9.0
Don't know/refused — 25.6

Percent response

effective in reducing the risk of infection is higher than the statewide proportion, but not significantly.

We also asked respondents to tell us where one could go to be tested for the AIDS virus. Just over 33 percent gave the emergency room, 31.8 percent named a private doctor, and 3.6 percent listed the health department. About 16.3 percent said they did not know. (See Exhibit 2–20.)

Cancer

Cancer accounts for one of every five deaths, may strike at any age, and does so with increasing frequency as people age. Overall U.S. costs for cancer were put at $72.5 billion in 1985. In 1990, it was estimated that cancer accounted for 11 percent of the total cost of disease. One in three people alive in 1990 will eventually have cancer.[14] It also appears that important strides in cancer cure and treatment are being made. Average survival time for people with cancer is increasing, and the death rate from all cancers declined between 1973 and 1987. Further, the potential for reducing the incidence of and mortality from cancer is great. More than 30 percent of cancer deaths are from cigarette smoking, and some studies indicate that as many as 35 percent of cancer deaths may be related to diet.[15] For this reason, increasing the public awareness of cancer symptoms will help reduce the incidence of the disease. We asked respondents to "please name any one of the seven warning signs of cancer." Results show the percentage of people who could name correctly at least one sign.

Our results showed that about 67.1 percent could correctly name at

EXHIBIT 2–20
Knowledge of AIDS Testing
Central Missouri, 1994

Test site

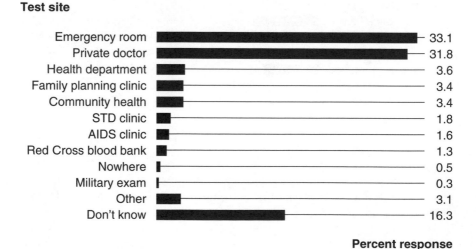

Test site	Percent response
Emergency room	33.1
Private doctor	31.8
Health department	3.6
Family planning clinic	3.4
Community health	3.4
STD clinic	1.8
AIDS clinic	1.6
Red Cross blood bank	1.3
Nowhere	0.5
Military exam	0.3
Other	3.1
Don't know	16.3

Percent response

least one warning sign. Thickening of or lumps in the breast was named by 28.7 percent; obvious changes in warts or moles was mentioned by 12.0 percent. About 24.6 percent could not name any sign. About 8.2 percent named a sign that was not a correct sign. (See Exhibit 2–21.)

Mammograms and Clinical Breast Exams

One study placed breast cancer as the second leading cancer death among women and indicated that about 1 woman in 10 will develop breast cancer in her lifetime. Controlled studies have further shown significant reduction in mortality due to breast cancer among women over the age of 50. Nevertheless, only 25 percent, nationwide, of women aged 50 or over had received clinical breast examinations or mammographies within the preceding two years in 1987.[16] Data from our study show that, of those women over the age of 55, 78.8 percent have had a mammogram and 91.1 percent have had a clinical breast exam. Within the past year, 50.0 percent

EXHIBIT 2-21
Seven Warning Signs of Cancer
Central Missouri, 1994

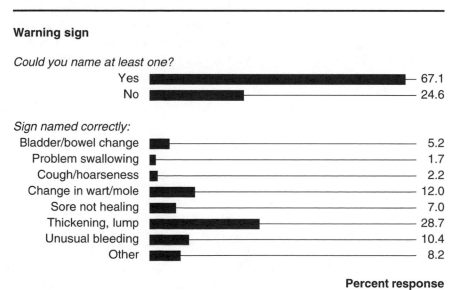

Warning sign

Could you name at least one?

Yes	67.1
No	24.6

Sign named correctly:

Bladder/bowel change	5.2
Problem swallowing	1.7
Cough/hoarseness	2.2
Change in wart/mole	12.0
Sore not healing	7.0
Thickening, lump	28.7
Unusual bleeding	10.4
Other	8.2

Percent response

have had a mammogram and 66.4 percent have had a clinical breast exam. Within the past two years, 67.8 percent have had a mammogram and 68.0 percent have had a clinical breast exam. The percentage of survey respondents over the age of 55 who report having had a mammogram within the past two years is significantly higher than the statewide figure.

Pap Tests

Cancer of the cervix is one of the most commonly occurring cancers for women. More than 50,000 cases are detected annually, and, of those women alive in 1990, 6,000 will die from cervical cancer. The Pap test greatly reduced the risk of death from cervical cancer, and one study concludes that the major cause of the decline in cervical cancer during the 1970s and 1980s is the widespread use of the Pap test. According to 1987 figures, 56 percent of women over the age of 28 received Pap tests every year. A recent study indicated that a "significant portion" of women are not receiving Pap tests regularly, and that those women at the greatest risk of death from cervical cancer are least likely to be screened.[17] About 9.6 percent of women over the age of 55 have never had a Pap test, but 55.5 percent have had a Pap test within the past year, and 67.1 percent have had a Pap test within the past two years. Further, 44.3 percent have had a mammogram but not within the past two years; 18.3 percent have had a clinical breast exam, but not within the past two years; and 26.4 percent have had a Pap test, but not within the past two years. The proportion of women over the age of 55 who report having had a Pap test within the past three years is significantly below the state average.

Analysis of Preventable Conditions

Recent research suggests that a sizable proportion of illnesses for which people seek medical attention can be substantially or entirely prevented through changes in behavior. One recent study found that as high as 40 percent of all illnesses are preventable. As argued in that study, "Understanding preventable conditions related to individual health behavioral patterns and their associated cost is one area that must be examined in developing a health assessment strategy."[18] (See Exhibit 2–22.)

Consistent with the analysis of preventable conditions presented in that study, we developed a list of 28 principal diagnoses identified by the Centers for Disease Control and Prevention. These conditions include heart attacks,

EXHIBIT 2–22
Assessment Area and State Data Compared

Indicator	Tri-County (percent)	State (percent)
Do not always wear a safety belt	34.1*	41.1
Sometimes, seldom, or never wears a safety belt	17.9*	25.6
Ever diagnosed with high blood pressure	27.8	24.5
Physically inactive	29.9	32.3
Currently trying to lose weight	33.3	N.A.
Smoked over 100 packs in a lifetime	50.7	26.6
Drinking over 60 drinks per month	2.0	2.4
Drinking 5 or more drinks on at least one occasion	19.7*	14.3
Had cholesterol checked less than 5 years ago	78.5*	64.4
Ever diagnosed with diabetes	11.6*	5.3
Without health insurance	21.6*	12.3
Agree that a person with AIDS can look well	77.7*	3.7
Say that a condom is very effective	24.8	20.5
Women over 55 who had mammogram within past 2 years	67.8*	54.4
Women over 55 who had Pap test within past 2 years	76.7*	85.5

* Denotes results more than 5.0 percentage points higher or lower than the comparable percentage for the state.

N.A. means not available.

Source: Data from the state taken from the Behavior Risk Factor Surveillance System available from the Missouri Department of Health.

hypertension, emphysema, alcoholism, obesity, and others. Examining discharge data for the assessment area, we determined that 990 of 2,609, or 37.9 percent, of all discharges for 1993 could have been substantially prevented.

ENDNOTES

1. *Healthy People 2000; National Health Promotion and Disease Prevention Objectives.* DHHS (PHS) Publication No. 91-50212. Washington, D.C.: U.S. Government Printing Office, 1991, p. 119.
2. *Healthy People 2000*, p. 282.
3. *Healthy People 2000*, pp. 398–99.

4. Harris, S.S.; C.J. Caspersen; G.H. DeFriese; and E.H. Estes. "Physical Activity Counseling for Healthy Adults as a Primary Preventative Intervention in a Clinical Setting." *Journal of the American Medical Association* (1989), 261:3590–3598.

Powell, K.E.; C.J. Caspersen; J.P. Koplan; and E.S. Ford. "Physical Activity and Chronic Disease." *American Journal of Clinical Nutrition* (1989) 49:999–1006.

Salonen, J.T.; P. Puska; and J. Tuomeliehto. "Physical Activity and Risk of Myocardial Infarction. Cerebral Stroke and Death: A Longitudinal Study in Eastern Finland." *American Journal of Epidemiology* (1982),115:526–537.

Cady, L.D.; E.P. Bischoff; E.R. O'Connell; P.C. Thomas; and J.H. Allan. "Strength and Fitness and Subsequent Back Injuries in Fire Fighters." *Journal of Occupational Medicine* (1979), 21:269–272.

Pfaffenbarger, R.S.; R.T. Hyde; A.L. Wing; and C.C. Hseih. "Physical Activity, All-Cause Mortality, and Longevity of College Alumni." *New England Journal of Medicine* (1986), 314:605–613.

Powell, K.E.; P.D. Thompson; C.J. Caspersen; and J.S. Kentrick. "Physical Activity and the Incidence of Coronary Heart Disease." *Annual Review of Public Health* (1987), 2:253–287.

Lewis, C.E., and K.B. Wells. "A Model for Predicting the Counseling Practices of Physicians." *Journal of General Internal Medicine* (1985), 1:14–19.

Leon, A.S.; J. Connett; D.R. Jacobs; and R. Raurama. "Leisure-time Physical Activity Levels and Risk of Coronary Heart Disease and Death." *Journal of the American Medical Association* (1987), 258:2388–2395.

Sallis, J.F.; W.L. Haskell; S.P. Fortmann; P.D. Wood; and K.M. Vranizan. "Moderate-intensity Physical Activity and Cardiovascular Risk Factors: The Stanford Five-City Project." *Preventive Medicine* (1986), 15:561–568.

All studies quoted in *Healthy People 2000*, p. 94.

5. *The Surgeon General's Report on Nutrition and Health.* DHHS (PHS) Pub. No. 88-50210. Washington, D.C.: U.S. Department of Health and Human Services, 1988.

6. *Healthy People 2000; National Health Promotion and Disease Prevention Objectives.* DHHS (PHS) Publication No. 91-50212. Washington, D.C.: U.S. Government Printing Office, 1991, p. 119.

7. *Reducing the Health Consequences of Smoking: Nicotine Addiction. A Report of the Surgeon General.* DHHS Pub. No. (CDC) 88-406. Washington, DC: U.S. Department of Health and Human Services, Office of Smoking and Health, 1988.

8. *Healthy People 2000*, p. 136.

9. Harwood, H.J.; D.M. Napolitana; P.L. Kristiansen; and J.J. Collins. *Economic Costs to Society of Alcohol and Drug Abuse and Mental Illness: 1980.* Research Triangle Park, NC: Research Triangle Institute, 1984.

Homberg, M.B. "Longitudinal Studies of Drug Abuse in a Fifteen-year-old Population." *ACTA Psychiatrica Scandinavia* (1985), 16:129–136.

Perrine, M.; R. Peck; and X. Fell. "Epidemiologic Perspectives on Drunk Driving." In *Surgeon General's Workshop on Drunk Driving: Background Papers*. Washington, D.C.: U.S. Department of Health and Human Services, 1989.

Clayton, R.R. "The Delinquency and Drug Use Relationship among Adolescents; A Critical Review." *NIDA Research Monograph 31*, in D.J. Lettieri and J. Ludford, eds., *Drug Abuse and the American Adolescent*. Washington, D.C.: U.S. Department of Health and Human Services, 1981; quoted in *Healthy People 2000*, p. 167.

10. National Center for Health Statistics. "Health United States, 1989." DHSS Pub. No. (PHS) 90-1232. Hyattsville, Md: US Department of Health and Human Services, 1990.

    National Heart, Lung and Blood Institute. "Hypertension Prevalence and the Status of Awareness, Treatment, and Control in the United States: Final Report of the Subcommittee on Definition and Prevalence of the 1984 Joint National Committee." *Hypertension* (1985), 7:457–468.

    In *Healthy People 2000*, p. 392.

11. American Diabetes Association Center for Economic Studies in Medicine. *Direct and Indirect Costs of Diabetes in the United States in 1987*. Alexandria, Va: The Association, 1988. In *Healthy People 2000*, p. 442.

12. *Healthy People 2000*, p. 460.

13. Hessol, N.A.; G.W. Rutherford; A.R. Lifson; et al. "The Natural History of HIV Infection in a Cohort of Homosexual and Bisexual Men: A Decade of Follow Up." *Abstract 4096: Proceedings of the IV International Conference on AIDS*. Stockholm, Sweden, June 14, 1988.

    Centers for Disease Control. *Morbidity and Mortality Weekly Report* (1990), 39(7):110–119.

    Centers for Disease Control. "Quarterly Report to the Domestic Policy Council on the Prevalence and the Rate of Spread of HIV and AIDS, United States." *Morbidity and Mortality Weekly Report* (1988), 37(14):223–226; as quoted in *Healthy People 2000*, p. 480.

14. American Cancer Society. *Cancer Facts and Figures—1989*. New York: The Society, 1990.

    Hodgson, T.A., and D.P. Rice. "Economics of Cancer in the United States." In D. Schottenfield, ed., *Cancer Epidemiology and Prevention*. Chapter 13 quoted in *Healthy People*, p. 416.

15. Eddy, D.M. "Setting Priorities for Cancer Control Programs." *Journal of the National Cancer Institute* (1986), 76:187–199.

    National Cancer Institute. "Cancer Control Objectives for the Nation; 1985–2000." *National Cancer Institute Monographs* (1986), vol. 2. DHHS Pub.

No. (NIH) 86–2880. Bethesda, Md: U.S. Department of Health and Human Services, 1986.

Ries, L.A.G.; B.F. Hankey.; and B.K. Edwards, eds. *Cancer Statistics Review 1973–1987*. NIH Pub. No. 90-2789. Bethesda, Md: U.S. Department of Health and Human Services, 1990.

In *Healthy People 2000*, p. 416.

16. American Cancer Society. *Cancer Facts and Figures*. National Cancer Institute and the National Center for Health Statistics. "1987 National Health Interview Survey, Cancer Control Supplement," unpublished.

Shapiro, S.; W. Venet; L. Strax; and R. Roeser. "Selection, Follow-up, and Analysis in the Health Insurance Plan Study: A Randomized Trial with Breast Cancer Screening." *National Cancer Institute Monographs* (1985), 67:65–74.

Tabar, L., et al. "Reduction in Mortality from Breast Cancer after Mass Screening with Mammography." *Lancet* (1985), 1:829–832.

Verbeek, A.L.M., et al. "Reduction of Breast Cancer Mortality through Mass Screening with Modern Mammography: First Results of the Nijmegan Project, 1975–1981." *Lancet* (1984), 1:1222–1224.

In *Healthy People 2000*, p. 420.

17. American Cancer Society. *Cancer Facts and Figures*. National Cancer Institute and the National Center for Health Statistics. "1987 National Health Interview Survey, Cancer Control Supplement," unpublished.

Shapiro, S.; W. Venet; L. Strax; and R. Roeser. "Selection, Follow-up, and Analysis in the Health Insurance Plan Study: A Randomized Trial with Breast Cancer Screening." *National Cancer Institute Monographs* (1985), 67:65–74.

Tabar, L., et al. "Reduction in Mortality from Breast Cancer after Mass Screening with Mammography." *Lancet* (1985), 1:829–832.

Verbeek, A.L.M., et al. "Reduction of Breast Cancer Mortality through Mass Screening with Modern Mammography: First Results of the Nijmegan Project, 1975–1981." *Lancet* (1984), 1:1222–1224.

International Agency for Research on Cancer Working Group on Evaluation of Cervical Cancer Screening Programs. "Screening for Squamous Cervical Cancer; Duration of Low Risk after Negative Results of Cervical Cytology and its Implications for Screening Policies." *British Medical Journal* (1986), 293:659–664.

In *Healthy People 2000*, pp. 421–422.

18. Engler, David. "A Health Status Assessment for Lifestyle Related Conditions." Presented in Columbus, Ohio, August 1994, Ohio Hospital Associations.

Chapter Three

Central Iowa

INTRODUCTION

Central County is located in central Iowa about 30 miles from Metro Area. As of the 1990 census, Central County was home to 74,000 households. Three hospitals serve the county: Central County Medical Center, a 216-bed hospital; Central City Hospital, a 36-bed facility; and Central County Hospital, a 122-bed facility. The county is also served by tertiary hospitals in Metro Area. Central City is the largest community in Central County.

HOW THE STUDY WAS CARRIED OUT

This study was conducted in two parts, the first part during spring 1994 and the second during late summer 1994. Our sources for this study were the 1990 federal census, a survey of community leaders, and a survey of the community. For the community leader survey, we focused only on Central County. For the survey of the community, we broadened our focus to bring in the opinions of people in a five-county area. Both surveys were conducted by telephone.

PROFILE OF CENTRAL COUNTY

A comparison of census data for Central County with comparable data for the state shows that Central County is relatively well off. Median age of Central County is 25.7 years, compared with 34.0 years for the state as a whole. About 6.3 percent of Central County residents are foreign-born, compared with 1.6 percent for the state. It has a lower unemployment rate than the state, 3.9 percent compared with 4.5 percent; its median household income is 100.2 percent of the state median income; and the percentage of families below the poverty level in Central County is 7.7, much lower than the 8.4 percent shown for Iowa as a whole.[1] Exhibit 3–1 compares these results for the county with the state.

EXHIBIT 3–1
Characteristics of Central County, Iowa

Characteristic	County	State
Mean number of persons per household	2.4	2.5
Age (in years):		
Percent under 5	5.9	7.0
Percent under 18	19.8	25.9
Percent 25 to 44	28.7	10.2
Percent 45 to 64	13.6	18.9
Percent 65 or over	9.6	15.3
Percent over 80	25.7	34.0
Percent foreign-born	6.3	1.6
Percent unemployed	3.9	4.5
Median household income in 1989 dollars	$26,668	$26,229
Percent of families below the poverty level	7.7	8.4

Services Available in Central County

Central County is well stocked with social services agencies. Even a cursory review of the *Directory of Health and Human Services for Residents of Central County*, published by United Way of Central County, suggests the range: general probation, educational, information, and referral services offered to the general population; services for AIDS victims and families; services to alcoholics and their families through Al-Anon, Alcoholics Anonymous, and Al-Ateen; services to the blind through the Lions Club; cancer education and assistance for victims and their families through the American Cancer Society; referrals, education, and advocacy to address child abuse through the Central Child Abuse registry, the Child Abuse Prevention and Education Council of Central County, and Child Safe; support and referral services for residential living situations and constructive community activities, and supervision of parole through the Division of Corrections; evaluation, assessment, and referral services through the Center for Addictions Recovery for those suffering from drug abuse; education, support, and advocacy services for the elderly; emergency services and low-priced or free merchandise availability through the American Red Cross, Community Thrift Shop, and the Bethesda Clothing Room; emergency shelter, outreach, information, referral, and advocacy as well as long-term healthcare for eligible Title-19 recipients, and financial assistance for the homeless and low-income residents; literacy services through the public library; information, advocacy, and referral services for the mentally ill through the Alliance for the Mentally Ill, Central Iowa Mental Health Center, and Cherokee Mental Health Institute; help for retarded and disabled persons through the Association for Retarded Citizens and the Central County Developmental Center; support for single parents through Parents without Partners and Sharing our Situation; financial and other assistance to veterans through the Commission on Veterans Affairs; support services for battered women through ACCESS; a variety of services to youth and families through a range of organizations, including Youth and Shelter Services, Inc., the Boy Scouts of America, Boys and Girls, Inc., Campfire, Children's Services in Central Iowa, and other organizations. A review of the service organizations available throughout the county substantiates this view. The primary needs in Central County lay in the need to coordinate the services available so they can work better for people. These are but a few of the services available to residents of Central County. Further, they include only those based in the county and serving the entire community. The list lengthens dramatically if organizations are included that serve the county but are based outside the county.

Pressing Health Concerns in Central County

To document and establish some priorities among competing health needs, we conducted a special survey of 47 social service agencies serving Central County, using our definition of "health" as the physical, emotional, and psychological well-being of people. In reading the material below, please remember that the words enclosed by quotations are accurate paraphrases, rather than precise transcriptions. We began each interview with the following question: "What would you say is the most pressing health problem or concern in Central County right now?" Responses were recorded, clarifying them when necessary.

The need most often identified was to provide medical services to low-income people, those eligible for medical assistance under Title 19, just above the cutoff line. "We need improved access and more financial assistance to those just above the poverty line to enable them to purchase medications," said one respondent. Another agreed that "accessibility to healthcare for low-income people" was a primary need, as well as "improved access for people with mental health and physical health needs who don't have enough money to get care." According to a third, the most urgent problem is "finding affordable healthcare. We try to make referrals outside [the agency], and we find that they have no insurance or benefits because they are unemployed or underemployed." Lack of care becomes a problem for a number of reasons, one of them "domestic violence, particularly for children and women." Children suffer because "lack of affordable and accessible healthcare" means that "families can afford both childcare and healthcare." In many cases, inadequate access to care requires "intervention with high-risk infants at the poverty level who experience family breakdown or stresses which place the family at risk." But it also means that a "major problem is coordinating services among numerous . . . providers. Lots of cracks in the system for people coming out of the hospital who need long-term services." And it also means "a dearth of services for seniors . . . to enable seniors to remain in their own homes as long as possible."

Current Efforts to Address the County's Needs

Next, we asked respondents to evaluate current efforts to meet or address the problems they identified. Most concurred that the needs are being met adequately. "Things are pretty much under control," noted one respondent; "we don't have any outbreak of disease or problems with our waste water." A representative of a mental health agency said, "The effort [to meet mental health needs] is adequate, so we don't have a crisis." And another agreed, pointing out that "we have a progressive county, with an array of services."

At the same time, the consensus was that there is a lot of room for improvement: "We are doing well in meeting basic needs, but we are not doing as much as we should be doing." And another reported that "there is no crisis, though things could be improved; we still have people who aren't being served." One area needing improvement was the coordination of mental health services: "We have made a start in addressing the better coordination of mental health services, but we need to move beyond the talking and planning stage to actually doing something." "We need more community collaboration to bring resources to bear on our problems," noted another, and a third said, "we need people to meet and talk together and examine the points where our agencies interface." Some areas identified for further work included: finding people who will go out into the community, drop-in centers, recruiting more doctors to rural areas, changing attitudes toward teens, efforts to combat child abuse, helping low-income and elderly people meet basic needs, better response to post-traumatic stress disorder, intervention in rural areas, combating stress and depression in teens, improving mental health services for the elderly, better facilities to treat Alzheimer's, more money for daycare, more help for people with their utility bills, improved detoxification services, dealing better with a lack of affordable housing, better emergency room care for the uninsured, meeting better the needs of the mentally ill, and better referrals of the homeless and uninsured.

The Role of the Community Hospital

Next, we asked respondents to name the organization or agency that would be best equipped to address community issues. Respondents gave a number of agencies they felt would be the appropriate agent of change in the county; but a strong consensus held that no one organization or agency was the appropriate change agent. Rather, there should be a group effort; a consortium of agencies should head the effort, with the local hospital, either alone or as a member of the consortium: "A group effort, not just one agency, which would include public health nurses, the hospital, mid-Iowa Community Action, C.A.P.E., and clinic pediatricians."

Today, the role of the community medical center is frequently controversial. Often it is seen as an obstacle blocking the road of community progress. We asked respondents their opinions about how well Central County Medical Center, the most important facility in the area, is doing to meet the overall health needs of the community. The medical center received about a B/B+, as high as any medical center we have studied. It was generally praised for its high level of medical care given to its patients: "They do a good job, and do a good job to help people financially, whenever they can; they help with rides and arrange rooms, and they go out of their way to help people in need." Another reported, "It is a good medical center; people feel good when they go there." A third said, "The medical center does very well, based on personal experience."

It received some criticism regarding its efforts to reach out to the community. "The medical center is fine for those who can afford it," said one critic; "I give it a B because of communication problems with the community." Said another: "The medical center is not a team player; it sets up programs that are duplicative." Another said, "They don't develop services in a 'planful' way. The medical center has expanded services into areas where other programs are already operating, and they have opened programs without documenting the need for them, when there was already a plethora of services available."

Key Health Needs in 10 Years

Respondents saw more of the same in the future. Any change needed was a stronger working partnership among agencies in the community: Central County Medical Center "will have to forge bonds and communicate better to move people through the system," said one respondent. Said another, "Central County Medical Center will have to expand to provide services to people who fall through the cracks." A third said, " Central County Medical Center will have to work with other agencies to provide alternative supportive services."

A second change was reform at the federal level: "We will need improved delivery of services to people who need them; action will have to come from the feds." Agreeing was a second respondent: "There will have to be reform at the national level; the local area can't make a dent in it." A third explained that "most of those in need are funded through Medicare; the whole reimbursement issue will have to be settled." A third group stressed that increases in funding were imperative: "we will need more money [to fund] low-cost child care, new psychiatric facilities, and services to seniors." Another noted that "breakdowns [in mental health] at early ages interrupt development of security, creating patterns of dysfunction and social problems; we need more advocacy, . . . good tools to identify risk, and we need money to use them." Finally, another argument stressed the role of education: "AIDS and smoking [will be major issues]; education will be important."

THE COMMUNITY'S PERSPECTIVE

So far we have examined the perceptions of social service agency representatives who sit close to the stage in Central County. Their perceptions have identified key health needs in the county. In any health needs assessment, however, it is important to bring the community's perspective, even if the community's approach is unsophisticated or even if its understanding of health issues could be more insightful. The health status of an area is affected when the local medical center does not have a close relationship with the people that it has been expected to serve. To bring the community's perspective to bear, we surveyed 418 households in Central County, and in the four counties that border it, West, North, South, and East counties, which were sampled in proportion to the number of households in each of the five counties. Random numbers in each of the counties were supplied by a firm that specializes in providing samples of random numbers to research companies and other organizations that conduct research over the telephone. Interviews were conducted from August 22 to September 7, 1994. Those interviewed were 18 years of age or older and involved in making the healthcare decisions for their households. All interviews were completed on weekday evenings and during the weekends to maximize interviewing efficiency. When, after an initial attempt, an interviewer did not complete an interview, two further attempts were made to contact the resident before substituting a new number.

For samples of this size, a maximum expected statistical error is +/– 5.0 percentage points at the 95 percent confidence level. This means that, if the study were replicated "N" times, the results for each item would be within 5.0 percentage points, high or low, of the observed result in 95 times out of 100 replications. Sampling is vulnerable to statistical error. Therefore, the reader should be careful when interpreting these findings. They are accurate, but precise only within the stated margins of error. One should interpret these results carefully and guard against attributing excess concreteness to differences among small subgroups. These subgroups may have larger margins of error associated with them.

DEMOGRAPHIC CHARACTERISTICS OF THE STUDY AREA

Sample Composition

Comparing the percentage breakdown of the sample with the area as a whole shows that West County was slightly undersampled and East County was slightly oversampled. However, given the level of precision of the study, the differences do not appear to be statistically significant. Further, to detect any differences due to sampling error, we weighted the sample so that the distribution of interviews would be present in the sample in the same proportion as households by county are represented in the survey area. The resulting analysis confirmed that there is no systematic bias introduced by deviation from the quotas. (See Exhibit 3–2.)

EXHIBIT 3–2
Sample Distribution and Household Composition

County	Percent of Households	Percent of Interviews	Sample Deviation
Central	40.1%	40.4%	0.3%
West	15.2	10.9	(4.3)
South	9.8	9.7	(0.1)
North	11.8	12.1	0.3
East	23.1	26.9	3.8
Total	100.0	100.0	0.0

About two-thirds of respondents were women, well in line with other studies, which show that in about two-thirds of households the healthcare decisions are made by women. The largest age group includes people from 45 to 64 years. Almost 9 in every 10 have lived in their current county five years or more, 3 out of every 4 for 10 years or more. (See Exhibit 3–3.)

Share of Mind

To begin each interview, we asked respondents, "Please name all the hospitals in your area that you can think of." We recorded the first three hospitals mentioned. Reviewing the distribution of mentions suggests that respondents included in their area West City on the west, Metro Area to the south, North City on the north, and East to the east. Further, it shows Central County Medical Center first, both in top-of-mind awareness and in total mentions. Three Metro Area hospitals follow, and East County Hospital is fifth. (See Exhibit 3–4.)

What People Are Looking for in Hospital Care

It was important to the management of Central County Medical Center to identify factors affecting the hospitals that people choose for medical care. First we asked, "When you are looking for the medical services that a hos-

EXHIBIT 3–3
Demographic Characteristics
Central Iowa, 1994

Characteristic

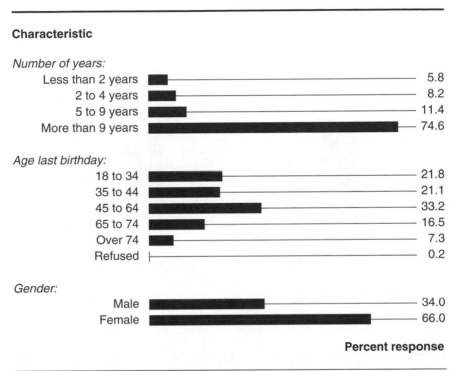

Number of years:

Less than 2 years	5.8
2 to 4 years	8.2
5 to 9 years	11.4
More than 9 years	74.6

Age last birthday:

18 to 34	21.8
35 to 44	21.1
45 to 64	33.2
65 to 74	16.5
Over 74	7.3
Refused	0.2

Gender:

Male	34.0
Female	66.0

Percent response

pital can provide, what factor is most important to you?" Possible choices included convenient parking, doctor's recommendation, ease of getting an appointment, good physicians, location, caring nurses, good reputation in the community, having local doctors, cost, modern equipment, recommendations of family and friends, short waiting time, well-trained specialists, or other factors. "Good doctors" was far and away the most often selected choice. Following in importance were the doctor's recommendation, good reputation in the community, and modern equipment. Cost was the least important. Exhibit 3–5 shows these results.

Next, we asked respondents to indicate the importance of selected hospital attributes on a scale of 1 to 10, where 10 is most important and 1 is least important. Attributes included quality of the medical staff, up-to-date equipment, quality of nursing care, availability of complete hospital services, caring attitude of employees, reputation in the community, cost,

EXHIBIT 3–4
Awareness of Area Hospitals
Central Iowa, 1994

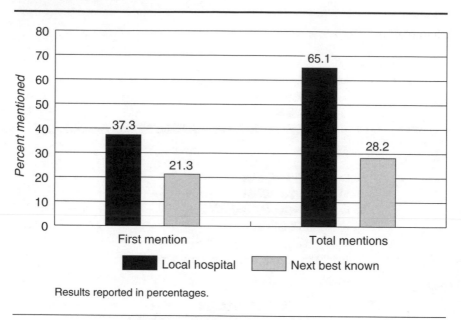

Results reported in percentages.

and advice of family and friends. The quality of the medical staff rated highest, having up-to-date equipment was second, and quality of nursing care was third most important. Advice from family and friends was rated least important, and the cost of care was almost as unimportant. (See Exhibit 3–6.)

Share of Outpatient, Inpatient, and Emergency Room Care

Exhibit 3–7 presents information about respondents' most recent visit to a hospital for emergency room, inpatient, and outpatient care. This exhibit shows that, within the past two years, about 30.8 percent of residents received inpatient care at a hospital, about 44.6 percent have received outpatient care at a hospital, and about 50.8 percent have received care at a hospital's emergency room. This situation is comparable with that in northern Missouri, and differs from patterns seen in northern Indiana.

EXHIBIT 3–5
Factors in Decisions
Central Iowa, 1994

Factor

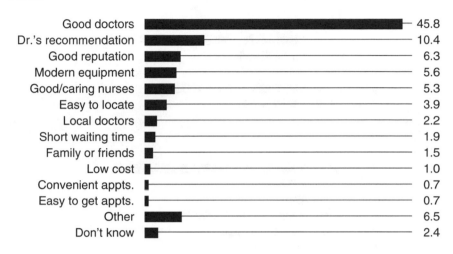

	Percent response
Good doctors	45.8
Dr.'s recommendation	10.4
Good reputation	6.3
Modern equipment	5.6
Good/caring nurses	5.3
Easy to locate	3.9
Local doctors	2.2
Short waiting time	1.9
Family or friends	1.5
Low cost	1.0
Convenient appts.	0.7
Easy to get appts.	0.7
Other	6.5
Don't know	2.4

EXHIBIT 3–6
Importance of Attributes
Central Iowa, 1994

Attribute

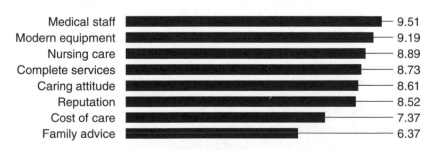

	Mean score
Medical staff	9.51
Modern equipment	9.19
Nursing care	8.89
Complete services	8.73
Caring attitude	8.61
Reputation	8.52
Cost of care	7.37
Family advice	6.37

EXHIBIT 3–7
Use of Inpatient, Outpatient and ER Care
Central Iowa, 1994

Service Used

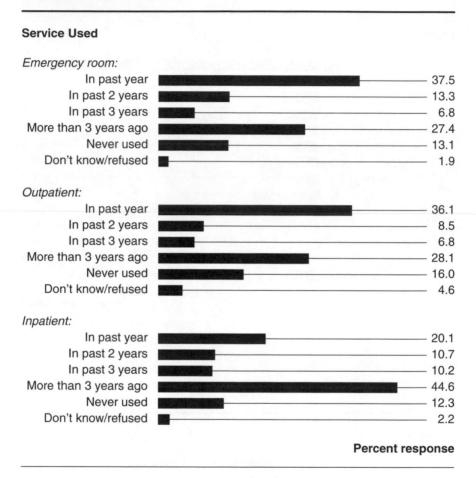

Emergency room:

In past year	37.5
In past 2 years	13.3
In past 3 years	6.8
More than 3 years ago	27.4
Never used	13.1
Don't know/refused	1.9

Outpatient:

In past year	36.1
In past 2 years	8.5
In past 3 years	6.8
More than 3 years ago	28.1
Never used	16.0
Don't know/refused	4.6

Inpatient:

In past year	20.1
In past 2 years	10.7
In past 3 years	10.2
More than 3 years ago	44.6
Never used	12.3
Don't know/refused	2.2

Percent response

Satisfaction with Care at Central County Medical Center

To measure the perceived quality of care at area hospitals, we asked those who had had direct experience with services at each hospital to give the hospital a grade, from A to F, as if they were in school, where an A is excellent and an F is failing. We then asked respondents who did not give the hospital an A what the hospital would have to have done to get an A. To calculate an average grade, we scored the grades so a 4 stands for an A and a 0 stands for an F. On the whole, hospital services received high marks, 3.25 (B+), for emergency care, 3.52 (B+/A–), for outpatient care, and 3.59 (B+/A–) for inpatient care. Central County Medical Center's marks were consistently above average: 3.73 for emergency room care, 3.61 for outpatient care, and 3.64 for inpatient care. (See Exhibit 3–8.)

Access to Medical Services

About 6.1 percent report having no health insurance. We asked each respondent: "Do you have a doctor that you see regularly when you need medical care?" Almost 2 in 10 do not have a physician they regard as a "regular." The phrase "regular physician" may not mean the same thing to everyone, but, however the term is defined, it is clear almost 20 percent of respondents do not have a physician to whom they feel they can turn when they need medical care. About 8 percent indicated they had delayed a medical visit because of cost during the past year.

EXHIBIT 3–8
Grades for Hospital Care
Central Iowa, 1994

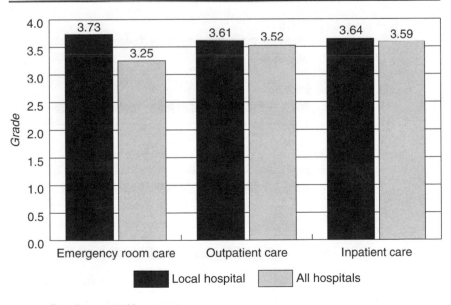

Results reported in percentages.

Next, we asked respondents: "Have you or has anyone in your family
had any difficulty finding a specialist in this area within the past two
years?" Only 6.1 percent, or 16 respondents, reported any problems at all
in finding a specialist. Those who did report problems said that they
hadn't known how to find one, or that they couldn't find a specialist in the
area. They reported having searched for a range of specialists, most frequently a neurologist, or another kind of specialist. (See Exhibit 3–9.)

Perceived Health Needs and Needed Medical Services

To gain some understanding of the perceived importance of specific
health problems and medical services, we asked respondents to point out
four types of services or problems. First, about the most important health
problems in their area, people gave as most important, 27.9 percent gave

EXHIBIT 3–9
Insurance and Physician Patterns
Central Iowa, 1994

Physician/insurance

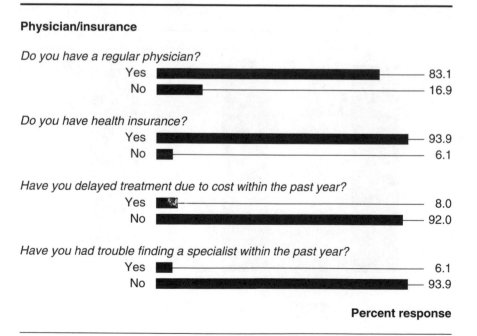

Do you have a regular physician?

Yes	83.1
No	16.9

Do you have health insurance?

Yes	93.9
No	6.1

Have you delayed treatment due to cost within the past year?

Yes	8.0
No	92.0

Have you had trouble finding a specialist within the past year?

Yes	6.1
No	93.9

Percent response

cancer; 13.7 listed heart problems; 10.3 percent listed care for the elderly; 9.3 percent mentioned the cost of healthcare. Other problems mentioned were lack of affordable insurance, drug and alcohol abuse, not enough doctors, general health problems, mental health and stress, back and knee problems, dialysis, overweight, HIV infections, and other problems. (See Exhibit 3–10.)

Next we asked people to tell us what health services were most needed in the area. Mentioned in response were: dialysis by 12.9 percent, more doctors or specialists by 11.8 percent, problems related to elderly care by 10.6 percent, cardiac care or specialists by 9.4 percent, public education about illness and prevention by 7.1 percent, cancer research and treatment by 5.9 percent. Other services needed in the area were: increased mental health services, more immunizations, better insurance coverage, drug abuse

EXHIBIT 3–10
Perceived Health Needs
Central Iowa, 1994

Perceived need

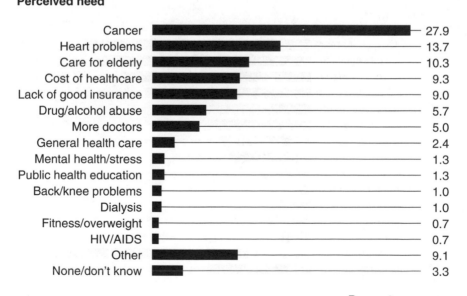

Cancer	27.9
Heart problems	13.7
Care for elderly	10.3
Cost of healthcare	9.3
Lack of good insurance	9.0
Drug/alcohol abuse	5.7
More doctors	5.0
General health care	2.4
Mental health/stress	1.3
Public health education	1.3
Back/knee problems	1.0
Dialysis	1.0
Fitness/overweight	0.7
HIV/AIDS	0.7
Other	9.1
None/don't know	3.3

Percent response

treatment, better emergency services, more or better free clinics, OB/GYN services, and a range of miscellaneous services. (See Exhibit 3–11.)

Third, what were the services people thought children were most likely to need? More pediatricians, mentioned by 15.6 percent; followed by more immunizations, mentioned by 9.1 percent; child or 24-hour wellness by another 9.1 percent; and child and domestic abuse services by 8.2 percent. Other services mentioned included cheap or free clinics, more doctors, educational programs, psychiatric services, cancer care, emergency room services, and a pediatric hospital ward. About 2.8 percent said "everything is covered," and about the same proportion said they didn't know. (See Exhibit 3–12.)

Finally, we wrap up this chapter by discussing what the elderly need. Most often mentioned was in-home care and services, by 19.2 percent.

EXHIBIT 3–11
Perception of Needed Services
Central Iowa, 1994

Perceived need

	Percent response
Dialysis center	12.9
More doctors/specialists	11.8
Care for elderly	10.6
Cardiac care	9.4
Public education	7.1
Cancer research	5.9
Mental health	5.3
Preventive health	4.7
Better insurance	2.9
Drug abuse treatment	2.5
Better ER	2.5
Free clinics	2.5
OB/GYN services	1.9
Other/misc.	14.6
None/don't know	5.9

EXHIBIT 3–12
Services Needed for Children
Central Iowa, 1994

Service

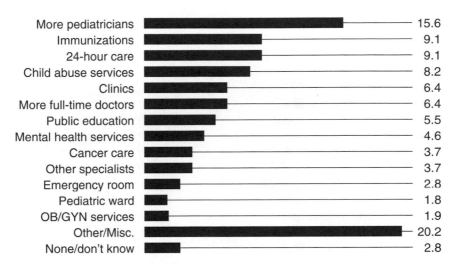

	Percent response
More pediatricians	15.6
Immunizations	9.1
24-hour care	9.1
Child abuse services	8.2
Clinics	6.4
More full-time doctors	6.4
Public education	5.5
Mental health services	4.6
Cancer care	3.7
Other specialists	3.7
Emergency room	2.8
Pediatric ward	1.8
OB/GYN services	1.9
Other/Misc.	20.2
None/don't know	2.8

Following were transportation, mentioned by 9.6 percent; lower-cost health-care by 7.1 percent; long-term care by 5.7 percent; Meals on Wheels by 3.2 percent; more attention paid to them; cardiac services, checkups, and educational services, mentioned by 2.6 percent; and a variety of other services. About 8 percent thought that all elderly people's needs were covered. (See Exhibit 3–13.)

ENDNOTE

1. See U. S. Department of the Census (1990): *Social and Economic Characteristics*, CP-2-17, Tables 1–3 and 6; *General Population Characteristics*, CP-1–17, Tables 1, 2, 5, and 54; *Summary and Housing Characteristics*, CPH 1–17, Tables 1, 2, 3, and 6.

EXHIBIT 3–13
Services Needed for Elderly
Central Iowa, 1994

Perceived need

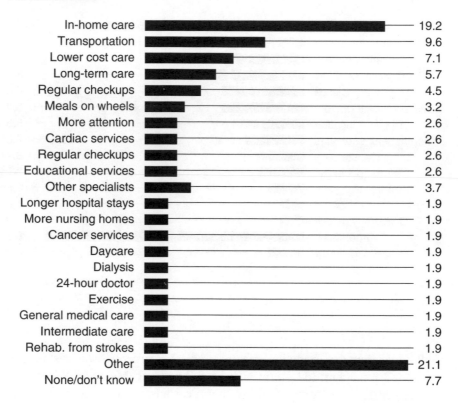

In-home care	19.2
Transportation	9.6
Lower cost care	7.1
Long-term care	5.7
Regular checkups	4.5
Meals on wheels	3.2
More attention	2.6
Cardiac services	2.6
Regular checkups	2.6
Educational services	2.6
Other specialists	3.7
Longer hospital stays	1.9
More nursing homes	1.9
Cancer services	1.9
Daycare	1.9
Dialysis	1.9
24-hour doctor	1.9
Exercise	1.9
General medical care	1.9
Intermediate care	1.9
Rehab. from strokes	1.9
Other	21.1
None/don't know	7.7

Percent response

Chapter Four

North County, Missouri, 1994

INTRODUCTION

North County, in northern Missouri, is largely agricultural. North County accounts for 10,536 people, about two-thirds of whom live in North City, North County's largest community. It is served primarily by a major route which runs north and south, to the west of North City. North County is served by North County Hospital, a small facility in North City, by community hospitals in adjacent counties, and by large tertiary hospitals in a major urban area nearby.

HOW THE STUDY WAS CARRIED OUT

This study was part of a larger effort carried out to assist the hospital in North County in recruiting physicians. To provide some guidance about what kinds of physicians to recruit, the study examined a whole range of data and studies, much of which is proprietary to the hospital and won't be covered here. Our sources for this study were federal census data, state discharge data supplied by the Health Industry Data Council, population projections supplied by the University of Missouri's demographic services center, surveyed community leaders, and surveyed people in the community. For analysis in this chapter, the "community" is defined as North County.

PROFILE OF NORTH COUNTY

Census data put the mean household income at $18,084, about $8,278 below the median household income for the state, and the percentage of families below the poverty line at 17, about 7 percentage points higher than the state. The North County educational level is somewhat higher than other counties in the area, but it is far behind the rest of the state in the percentage of high school graduates enrolled in college. (See Exhibit 4–1.)

Growth projections available from the University of Missouri indicated a decline in population of between 0.3 percent and 4.6 percent over the next 20 years. Most of the decline will come at the young and older end of the age spectrum, because outmigration will offset the gains in births over deaths. The remaining population will be more concentrated in the 40 to 60 age cohort than at present. Some new industrial expansion is developing near the county, but it probably will not do much to overcome the long-term population decline projected by state of Missouri demographers.

Health Status Indicators

In 1990, the state of Missouri's Center for Health Statistics published health status indicators. A series of volumes presented data on a range of indicators for the county, the region, and the state. I have extracted those data that were statistically above or below the statewide ratio and presented them in Exhibit 4–2. Except where indicated, all figures are ratios expressed as the number of cases per 100,000 population.

Of 82 health status indicators collected by the state of Missouri, North County deviates significantly from the state average on 15. Even though I have reproduced them here, the numbers should be interpreted with caution: some data are more than 10 years old, some are incomplete, and some are based on a prevalence that makes them unreliable.

EXHIBIT 4–1
Social and Economic Characteristics of North County, Missouri

Characteristic	County	State
Median age	40	34
Percent under 18 years old	24	25
Percent over 65 years old	22	15
Median household income	$18,084	$26,362
Percent of families below poverty line	17	10
High school dropout ratio	8	11
Percent 18–35 enrolled in college	31	34

EXHIBIT 4–2
Health Status Indicators for North County and Missouri

Indicator	County	State
Percent of population over 65 on Medicaid	12	9
Deaths from heart disease	2,765	2,081
Deaths from malignant neoplasms	818	1,007
Deaths from cerebrovascular disease	576	481
Percent clients of home health agencies	8	10
EMS runs of 30 minutes or more	10	44
Medicaid recipients in:		
Intermediate care facilities	50	40
Long-term and alternative care	54	31
Percent of hospital discharges outside RPG	19	14
Average length of stay (days)	7	9
Live births	51	64
Births out of wedlock	10	23
Abortions	96	249
Prenatal WIC participants	42	22
Premature births	7	9

SOCIAL SERVICE INVENTORY

To evaluate currently available services, and to address community health and social welfare issues, we surveyed representatives of community organizations and spokespersons for 17 agencies currently working in North County and the surrounding area. A directory of social service agencies and other directories provided the names and phone numbers. These sources document that a wide range of resources is available to North County: educational and nutritional services for preschool children through the Head Start program in North City; mental health services for the North City community through the Northern Missouri Mental Health Center; enhanced mental and physical well-being of children under five years old through the programs of the Kiwanis Club; coordinated efforts to enhance the social and spiritual health of residents, and some financial assistance, through the Ministerial Alliance; assistance with promoting vision and preventing blindness through the Lions Club; programs to give residents access to assistance with human resources and living skills through the local conservation and development council; home meal delivery and other programs to assist the elderly in living in their homes run by the North County Council on Aging; nursing home services from convalescent care to hospice services at Manor Care Center and Nursing Home; programs to recruit, train, and educate health professionals in the northern Missouri area through the Health Education Center; two-year vocational educational programs in nursing and other areas of health from the North City Community College in North City; protective services and other programs available for the elderly through the Division of Aging; programs to promote good community health, freedom from communicable diseases, good public school health, food, and nutrition through the North County Health Department; public assistance, AFDC, food stamps, Medicaid reimbursement for children and the elderly, blind care, and child care from the Division of Family Services; employment assistance and training from the Area Job Training Partnership Administration; home health and other services through Services for Older Americans, Inc.; employment and training for people aged 55 or over from Green Thumb; services and law enforcement for youth from the 3rd Judicial Circuit Juvenile Court; counseling and other social services for battered women and abused children at the Women and Children's Shelter in North City; programs designed to eliminate cancer as a major health problem by the American Cancer Society chapter; assistance for individuals in need gained from Church Women United; agricultural and educational programs and assistance through the University of Missouri Extension; programs and services to improve the business climate in North County through the North City Area Chamber of Commerce; and mental health services through the North County Learning Center.

HEALTH AND SOCIAL WELFARE ISSUES IN NORTH COUNTY

Most Pressing Health Problems

To identify the most pressing problems, issues, and concerns, I interviewed representatives of 25 area agencies and organizations. The interview lasted on average from 9 to 15 minutes and was qualitative in nature. Some were briefer than others: my shortest conversation lasted 6 minutes, my longest lasted 20 minutes. After gathering some background information on the person I was interviewing and on the agency that person represented, I indicated our starting point: "The point of our study is to gain your perspective on the most important health issues or concerns in North County. . . . We are interested in your perspective as a person who is active in the affairs of North County. And we are looking at health in a very broad context, one that incorporates environmental, emotional, and psychological well-being in addition to the absence of disease. . . . From this perspective, then, what would you say is the most pressing health problem, issue, or concern in North County right now?" Respondents were left to answer whatever came to mind and were probed until they provided up to three responses.

Fourteen of the 25 respondents mentioned the need for more doctors. Further, 9 of the 14 respondents who identified the need for more doctors mentioned it first. "We need more GPs in North County," said one respondent; "we're in a growth situation with new industry moving in." Another explained more fully: "We have a high ratio of population to doctors. One is moving away to Princeton. The hospital is doing all it can to bring in specialists, but having enough skilled doctors is the biggest problem. There is a strong feeling across the area that for skilled care, people have to go outside the area, 'to the city.'"

Eight of the 25 respondents identified the need to deliver babies as a key health need. One mentioned it first, six mentioned it second, and one mentioned it third. "The local hospital needs to deliver babies," said one respondent; "right now they can't be born there." Another expressed his dismay that "no one delivers babies any more. I don't know why. The money is there, as is the need for it. But they aren't."

Seven respondents noted transportation difficulties. The Organized Alternative Transportation Program, based in St. Joseph, Missouri, has one bus which operates within North County itself, but makes only one run per month out of the area. For travel to the city for tests or treatment, area residents must rely on friends, relatives, or volunteers from a church or voluntary service organization.

Six respondents noted the lack of or inadequacy of insurance in the area. One said: "People lack funds. They can't even go to the doctor for maintenance or for regular checkups." Another explained that "medicine is too expensive and not covered, so people mess [sic] with their doses." Others cited high incidence of cancer, children's poor health, limited services for the elderly, inadequate healthcare locally, and general health problems, such as limited training funds, lack of physical or speech therapy, loneliness, nutrition problems, long waits in the emergency room, alcohol and drug abuse among teens, and other problems. (See Exhibit 4–3.)

Current Efforts to Meet the Need

Next, I asked respondents to evaluate current efforts to meet or address the problems they identified in the previous question. Respondents quite candidly offered their evaluation of current efforts. Here I have included discussion of the top three needs identified: more doctors, to deliver babies locally, and better transportation.

Leaders in the community were quite aware of the hospital's attempts to recruit physicians who can deliver babies. The consensus was that, while the effort was not bearing fruit, the effort was being made. According to one respondent, "The new administrator is trying to get additional physicians in the area. I don't know whether they are trying the right methods, and I don't know how effective they are being." According to another respondent, "Some attempt is being made to recruit, and I think the effort is sufficient." A third had a different assessment: "The hospital is trying to recruit doctors.

EXHIBIT 4–3
Community Leaders' Concerns
North County, Missouri, 1994

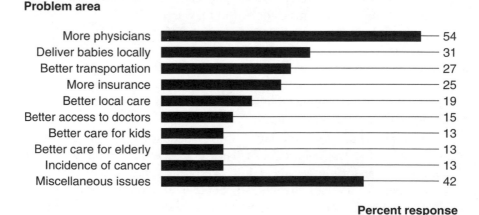

Problem area

More physicians	54
Deliver babies locally	31
Better transportation	27
More insurance	25
Better local care	19
Better access to doctors	15
Better care for kids	13
Better care for elderly	13
Incidence of cancer	13
Miscellaneous issues	42

Percent response

They are trying to take it on themselves. A firm didn't find any doctors. The most recent doctor came here because she grew up in North City. I don't know what else they could do, but I don't think they are being very effective." According to a fourth: "There are several recruitment efforts underway, [but] I don't know whether they are getting an OB. I don't know; I don't think they are being very effective." A fifth: "The hospital is trying to recruit new doctors; they're not very effective. There aren't any new ones yet [because] it is hard to recruit in rural areas." A sixth agreed that "the hospital is encouraging physicians, but it is hard to find doctors to come into rural areas; the hospital is being as effective as it can be, certainly better than it used to be." A seventh said, "The hospital does what it can to bring in prospects, [but] I don't know how well they are doing." An eighth thought the community should back up the hospital's efforts more enthusiastically: "[It] is doing whatever it can; I don't know what more they can do; the community could be more active; they should work with the hospital more." A ninth was more critical of the board: "The hospital administrator is encouraging physicians; he is working hard to bring in physicians, but he isn't getting cooperation from the board." A tenth respondent laid the blame at the feet of the medical community: "The doctors at the hospital are trying to recruit physicians. I don't know how effective they are. The problem needs to be addressed by the medical community."

The need for better transportation was a major area identified. It is particularly important in North County, because the area is sparsely populated and a person can only with difficulty get to the hospital in North City or to the larger tertiary facilities in Kansas City. Respondents felt that efforts to improve transportation in the county are insufficient, and they see the primary need in lack of funding. Respondents' comments reflected a sense of strong frustration concerning efforts to improve the area's transportation problems. Here is one example: "I don't know what can be done locally; there is talk about the need for transportation, especially for young mothers without cars; there's no funding for transportation; it's very frustrating, being not very effective." Another noted that the local bus service "works somewhat effectively to 'haul' people, but if they need radiation treatment, they have to rely on the family. The need is not being addressed; it's strictly a family responsibility. The local bus service is working O.K. locally, but not outside." According to a third, "There is funding for [the bus service], but they're barely touching the problem."

There was a strong sentiment in favor of a consortium or group effort made up of service organizations, government agencies, and service clubs.

"Trying to leave it up to one organization is wrong. It needs to be addressed by the whole community." Three thought their own organization to be more appropriate, and three thought the best-equipped organizations to meet community needs are the universities and the medical communities.

Key Health Needs in 10 Years

Nine see the growth in elderly residents as the most important problem in 10 years. Right behind is a group of eight respondents who think the physician shortage will still be a problem in 10 years. Three respondents think that in 10 years AIDS will be a key health problem; three think that the rising cost of health coverage will be a key problem; and seven cited other problems such as cancer, homelessness, children's safety, transportation, more AODA, and other factors.

HEALTH PRACTICES AND PATTERNS IN NORTH COUNTY

Introduction

In this section of the chapter, I present information from a community survey conducted in North County. The survey focused on health-related behaviors affecting the health status of the community in North County. The survey was conducted by telephone from March 10 to March 15, 1994. Data were collected on 207 households and are precise with a margin of error of 8.5 percent, high or low, at the 95 percent level of confidence. This means, assuming we find a result of 50 percent on a given question, that, if we were to replicate the study "N" times, we would find that result falling between 41.5 percent and 58.5 percent 95 times out of every 100 replications.

Characteristics of the Sample

First, let's look at the demographic characteristics of the sample, each of which was in the right proportion as shown by the census, taking into consideration sample variation. About 80 percent had lived in the area 10 or more years; ages were rather evenly distributed across the sample; and

71 percent were female, about the same proportion that normally participate in surveys. (See Exhibit 4–4.)

Use of Hospital Care

Next, let's look at the use of care at a hospital. Consistent with national
trends, outpatient use far outstripped inpatient use. Within the past two
years, 41 percent had been admitted to a hospital as an inpatient; 82 percent

EXHIBIT 4–4
Residence, Age, and Gender
North County, Missouri, 1994

Characteristic

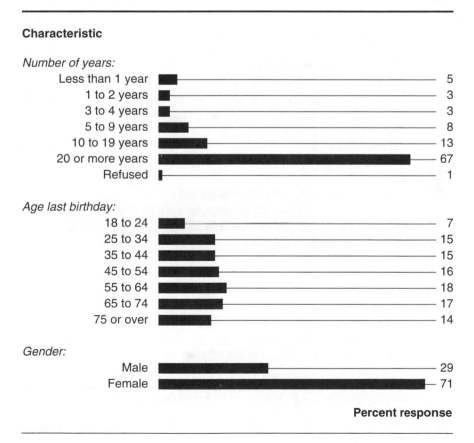

Number of years:

Less than 1 year	5
1 to 2 years	3
3 to 4 years	3
5 to 9 years	8
10 to 19 years	13
20 or more years	67
Refused	1

Age last birthday:

18 to 24	7
25 to 34	15
35 to 44	15
45 to 54	16
55 to 64	18
65 to 74	17
75 or over	14

Gender:

| Male | 29 |
| Female | 71 |

Percent response

had used a hospital as an outpatient, and 36 percent had used a hospital's emergency room. (See Exhibit 4–5.)

Regular Doctor

In North County, 86 percent of respondents have a doctor they consider a "regular" doctor. About 23 percent reported trouble finding a physician, primarily because they couldn't get a convenient appointment or because

EXHIBIT 4–5
Inpatient, Outpatient, and ER Care
North County, Missouri, 1994

Type of care

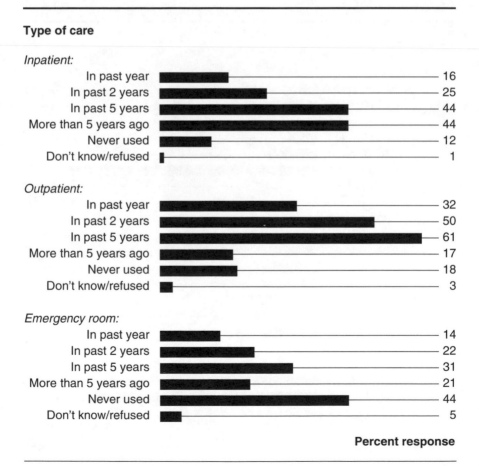

Inpatient:	
In past year	16
In past 2 years	25
In past 5 years	44
More than 5 years ago	44
Never used	12
Don't know/refused	1

Outpatient:	
In past year	32
In past 2 years	50
In past 5 years	61
More than 5 years ago	17
Never used	18
Don't know/refused	3

Emergency room:	
In past year	14
In past 2 years	22
In past 5 years	31
More than 5 years ago	21
Never used	44
Don't know/refused	5

Percent response

the physicians were not taking on new patients. About 17 percent reported having trouble finding a specialist, most of the time because there wasn't a specialist within the area. These findings illustrate the need for more physicians in the North County area. Community leaders noted it as a need; consumers found it hard to find a physician or specialist. (See Exhibit 4–6.)

Health Insurance

Lack of health insurance is a problem in North County; 17 percent have no health insurance of any kind. Even those with health insurance, however, were not fully insured. Those who had health insurance were asked

EXHIBIT 4–6
Physician Patterns
North County, Missouri, 1994

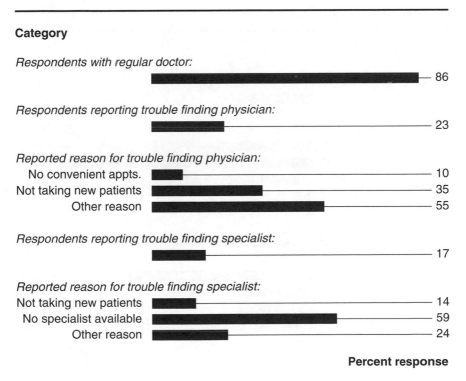

Category

Respondents with regular doctor:
86

Respondents reporting trouble finding physician:
23

Reported reason for trouble finding physician:
No convenient appts. — 10
Not taking new patients — 35
Other reason — 55

Respondents reporting trouble finding specialist:
17

Reported reason for trouble finding specialist:
Not taking new patients — 14
No specialist available — 59
Other reason — 24

Percent response

to tell us how much of their costs were covered. About 22 percent indicated their insurance did not cover all expenses, and 15 percent reported that their health insurance did not cover all expenses for visits to doctors. The degree of underinsurance, the extent to which insurance pays less than all costs, was quite high. (See Exhibit 4–7.)

Most Pressing Health Need

We asked North County residents to indicate the most pressing health needs in their community. They focused on the same health needs as the community leaders had. Four items topped the list: more or better doctors was chosen by 44 percent, high cost of healthcare by 19 percent, cancer by 6 percent, and the need for better facilities by 5 percent. (See Exhibit 4–8.)

EXHIBIT 4–7
Health Insurance Data
North County, Missouri, 1994

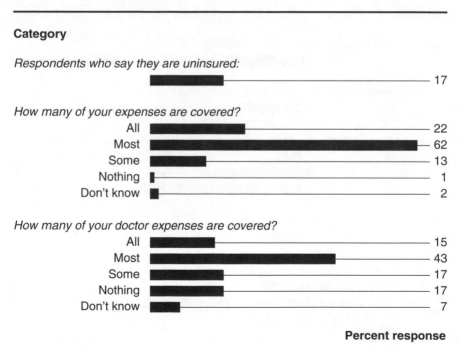

Category

Respondents who say they are uninsured:
17

How many of your expenses are covered?
All	22
Most	62
Some	13
Nothing	1
Don't know	2

How many of your doctor expenses are covered?
All	15
Most	43
Some	17
Nothing	17
Don't know	7

Percent response

EXHIBIT 4–8
Perception of Key Needs
Northern Missouri, 1994

Perceived need

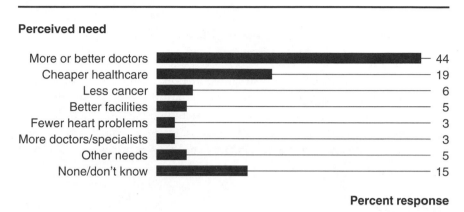

	Percent response
More or better doctors	44
Cheaper healthcare	19
Less cancer	6
Better facilities	5
Fewer heart problems	3
More doctors/specialists	3
Other needs	5
None/don't know	15

Health-Related Behaviors

To complete the survey, we asked respondents about behaviors that affect the health status of the community. This information is key for community health planning because it offers targets that can guide health planners' efforts. Our study in North County was not as extensive as in some other areas, but analyses of these data show what can be done with such data when examined in a comparative framework. Questions for this section of the survey were taken from the behavioral risk factor survey conducted by the Centers for Disease Control and Prevention conducted monthly through the Missouri Department of Health. Results for North County are directly comparable with data taken statewide, and we can position North County vis-à-vis the state on each of the questions asked on the survey.

High Blood Pressure

First, we asked respondents when was the last time they had had their blood pressure taken by a doctor, nurse, or other healthcare professional. About 79 percent had had their blood pressure taken during the past six months, 89 percent during the past year, and 93 percent during the past two years. Nearly 26 percent had been told that they had high blood pressure, 72 percent were told more than once, and 72 percent of those who were told more than once were not taking medication. (See Exhibit 4–9.)

Exercise, Smoking, and Consumption of Alcohol

About 26 percent of respondents do not engage in any form of exercise, such as running, swimming, calisthenics, or golf. About 38 percent have smoked at least 100 cigarettes in their lives, and of these, 56 percent currently smoke, and 36 percent smoke more than one pack of cigarettes per day. About 15 percent drink alcoholic beverages in a typical week, most often one day or less per week. On a typical day, those who drink will have one or two. (See Exhibit 4–10.)

EXHIBIT 4–9
Blood Pressure Data
North County, Missouri, 1994

Indicator

Last check by healthcare professional:

Past 6 months	79
Past year	89
Past 2 years	93
Past 5 years	97
More than 5 years ago	1
Never	1
Don't know	1

Respondents told they have high blood pressure: 26

Respondents told more than once they have high blood pressure: 72

Respondents told they have high blood pressure and not taking meds for same: 72

Percent response

Percentages may not total 100 due to multiple responses.

EXHIBIT 4–10
Exercise, Smoking, and Alcohol
North County, Missouri, 1994

Indicator

Respondents who do not participate in any form of exercise:

——————————————————————— 26

Respondents who have smoked more than 100 cigarettes in their lives:

——————————————————————— 38

Respondents who have quit smoking:

——————————————————————— 44

Respondents who smoke more than one pack a day:

——————————————————————— 36

Respondents who drink alcoholic beverages in a typical week:

——————————————————————— 15

Percent response

Cholesterol and Diabetes

About 20 percent of respondents have never had their blood cholesterol checked, and 5 percent have not checked their cholesterol within the past five years. About 25 percent have never been tested for diabetes; 5 percent were checked more than five years ago, and 16 percent do not remember. (See Exhibit 4–11.)

Women's Health Issues

About 49 percent of the women surveyed have never had a mammogram; of those who have had a mammogram, 17 percent had not had one within the past five years. About 13 percent of women surveyed have never had a clinical breast exam. Of those who have had one, 15 percent have not had one within the past year. About 13 percent of women have never had a Pap test; of those who have had one, 20 percent have not had one within the past five years. (See Exhibit 4–12.)

EXHIBIT 4–11
Cholesterol and Diabetes
North County, Missouri, 1994

Indicator

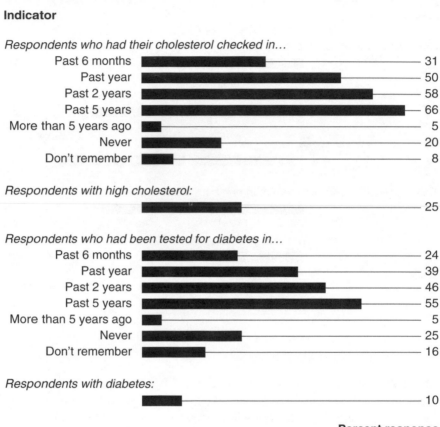

Respondents who had their cholesterol checked in...

Past 6 months	31
Past year	50
Past 2 years	58
Past 5 years	66
More than 5 years ago	5
Never	20
Don't remember	8

Respondents with high cholesterol:

25

Respondents who had been tested for diabetes in...

Past 6 months	24
Past year	39
Past 2 years	46
Past 5 years	55
More than 5 years ago	5
Never	25
Don't remember	16

Respondents with diabetes:

10

Percent response

Percentages may not total 100 due to multiple responses.

Share of Mind

Finally, an important health status indicator is the awareness of and usage of the local hospital. The hospital is an important actor in the healthcare drama of local communities, and these two factors—awareness and usage—are important indicators of the health of a community. In a healthy community, people are aware of and are proud of their hospital. Respon-

EXHIBIT 4–12
Women's Health Issues
North County, Missouri, 1994

Indicator

Mammograms:

Never had one	49
In past year	44
In past 2 years	53
In past 5 years	83
More than 5 years ago	17

Clincal exams:

Never had one	13
In past year	58
In past 2 years	71
In past 3 years	79
In past 5 years	85
More than 5 years ago	15

Pap tests:

In past year	47
In past 2 years	57
In past 3 years	70
In past 5 years	78
More than 5 years ago	20

Percent response

Percentages may not total 100 due to multiple responses.

dents were first asked to name all the hospitals they could think of in their area. Interviewers recorded the first three hospitals they mentioned. We calculated the number of times each hospital was mentioned and came up with both a top-of-mind awareness measure, the proportion of people who mentioned each hospital first, and a total awareness figure, the total number of times a hospital was mentioned either first, second, or third, divided by the total number of respondents. Top-of-mind awareness for North County Hospital was 71.0 percent, and total awareness was 92 percent.

These figures are very high for such a community as North County. Then, using discharge statistics for the county and for the hospital, I reviewed the percentage of the local hospital's patients and the county they came from, and the proportion of the county that used each hospital. North County Hospital showed a 62 percent share of all discharges from North County; and of all patients discharged from North County Hospital, 72 percent came from North County. These figures are quite acceptable for a community of this type. (See Exhibit 4–13.)

EXHIBIT 4–13
Awareness of Local Hospital
North County, Missouri, 1994

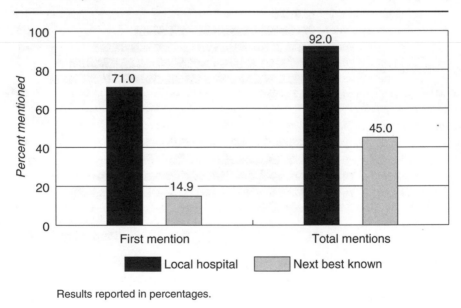

Results reported in percentages.

Chapter Five

North County, Indiana

INTRODUCTION

North County lies in northern Indiana about 30 miles from large metropolitan areas on the northeast, 45 miles from a large metropolitan area on the northwest, and about 110 miles from a large metropolitan area on the south. North County covers about 313 square miles and, according to the 1990 census, has a population of 22,751. North County's largest community and county seat, North City, has a population of 7,437. The area was originally settled in the nineteenth century by migrants from Ohio and New England, as well as by people moving northward out of Kentucky and Tennessee. It has a growing industrial base, but 88.5 percent of the county is still classified as agricultural by the Federal Bureau of the Census.

The county is served by a major four-lane highway that runs from northern Illinois through Chicago's eastern suburbs, southeast across Indiana, then on to the east. A straight two-lane road runs from the south through the area to the north. The area is served by North County Memorial Hospital, a 34-bed community hospital located in North City, five community hospitals within an easy drive of Knox, and major urban tertiary hospitals.

According to 1990 census figures, one household in eight is below the poverty level, and just over 8 percent of the labor force is unemployed. Most jobs require little skill, and there are few employment opportunities within the county.

HOW THE STUDY WAS CARRIED OUT

I conducted this study in the summer of 1993 to help North County Memorial Hospital understand its position in the community, to define the range of health problems that need to be addressed, and to pinpoint the key health needs of the area. The results of the study were designed to help the hospital develop an agenda for action.

There were three parts of the study. First, I reviewed data from the census and from a health assessment completed in 1989 by the Indiana Department of Health. Next, I conducted a survey of representatives of social service and governmental agencies providing service to the county. Interviewees represented the following agencies: Planned Parenthood of Northwest/Northeast Indiana; Indiana Work Force Development Services; VNA Home Care Services; Kiwanis Club; North County Council on Aging; state welfare department; Porter Starke Counseling Services; Interventions for Youth; Home Health Care Services; North County WIC Program; Community Guidance for Youth; North County Probation Department; the Disabled Services Association; and Knox Community School Corporation. Finally, I conducted a consumer opinion survey of the community. Analysis of the survey was based on 300 completed interviews. Most of the questions on the survey asked people's opinions of the local hospital and will not be covered in this book. However, several questions did solicit public input on health needs, and I have included some discussion of the results. Our work also included several recommendations made to the local hospital, and those have also been left out of this account. (See Exhibit 5–1.)

RESULTS FROM THE 1990 FEDERAL CENSUS

EXHIBIT 5–1
Census Data from North County Compared with the State of Indiana

Characteristic	County	State
Median household size	2.45	2.61
Percent of women over 65 living alone	12.0	8.1
Age distribution:		
Percent under 5	6.1	7.2
Percent under 18	23.2	26.3
Percent 18 to 24	14.9	10.9
Percent 25 to 44	26.9	31.3
Percent 45 to 64	19.0	19.0
Percent 65 or older	16.0	12.6
Percent 80 or older	4.2	2.9
Median age	33.5	32.8
Percent of persons, aged 16–19, not in high school and not graduated	6.4	11.4

EXHIBIT 5–1 continued

Percent of persons, aged 18–24, enrolled in college	63.6	34.6
Percent unemployed	6.7	5.7`
Percent of families for whom poverty status is determined	11.4	7.9
Median household income*	$27,732	$34,082

* U.S. Department of the Census, 1990: *Social and Economic Characteristics*, vol. CP-2-6, Tables 1–3; *General Population Characteristics*, vol. CP-1-6, Tables 1 and 2.

RESULTS FROM THE HEALTH DEPARTMENT SURVEY

In 1989, the Indiana Department of Health conducted a health needs assessment of each county in Indiana. The study used 39 indicators to measure the health status of each county. The indicators fell into five age groups: infants less than one year old; children 1–14 years old; adolescents and young adults; adults of all ages; and adults aged 65 years or older. North County met or exceeded minimum criteria of adequacy on only 10 indicators. Of the 39 indicators, the county bettered the standard on only 10 indicators. You can see the Indiana Health Department results listed in Exhibit 5–2.

EXHIBIT 5–2
Healthcare Adequacy in North County, Indiana

Criteria	Adequacy Standard*	Meets/Exceeds Standard
Infants, less than 1 year:		
Infant mortality rate	9 deaths	No
Low birth weight (less than 5.5 pounds)	50 births	No
Nonwhite low birth rate	9 births	No
Women with prenatal care	90 in first trimester	No
Children, 1–14 years:		
Overall death rate, 1–4 years	42 deaths	No
Overall death rate, 1–14 years	29 deaths	No
Indigenous measles	0	Yes
Immunity levels	970	Yes
Child abuse cases	2.21 cases	No
Child neglect cases	2.18 cases	No

EXHIBIT 5–2 continued

Licensed child care centers meet current health and nutrition standards	1,000	Yes
Live births in females, 10–14	0	Yes
Pregnancy in females, 15–19	58	No
Adolescents and young adults:		
Overall death rate, 15–24	8.54	No
Unintentional death rate, 15–24	4.5	No
Live births in females, 15–19	44 births	No
Pregnancy in females, 15–19	58	No
Gonorrhea	0.068	Yes
Syphilis	0.080	No
Adults, all ages:		
Overall death rate	88.73 deaths	No
Unintentional death rate	3.5 deaths	No
Heart disease rate	31.0 cases	No
Cerebrovascular disease	6.5 deaths	No
Cancer death rate	21.0 deaths	No
Diabetes death rate	1.5 deaths	Yes
Community water system	Fluoridation, 1 part per million	No
Homicide death rate	0.51 deaths	No
Suicide death rate	1.16 deaths	No
Older adults, over 64 years:		
Adult daycare program	1 in place	No
Alzheimer's support group	1 in place	Yes
Older adult nursing program	1 in place	Yes
Respite care support services	1 in place	No
Endangered adults	27	No
Sanitarian on staff	1 in place	No
RN per 15,000 population	1	No
Restaurant inspections	Twice a year	Yes
Nutrition	50 percent of population served by WIC	Yes
PCP licensed	1 per 3,500 population	Yes

* Except where indicated, all figures are expressed per 1,000.

COMMUNITY LEADER SURVEY

The study addressed the following eight questions: (1) What is the community's most pressing health problem? (2) What groups in the community are currently underserved? (3) How is the need currently being met? (4) Who is currently working to meet it? (5) How adequately is the need being met? (6) Who should take the lead role in addressing it? (7) What groups should be mobilized in an effort to meet this need? and (8) How should the hospital bring various groups into the process?

We interviewed representatives of 12 agencies during August 1993. Data were collected through a qualitative interview lasting, on average, about 20 minutes. Because the interview was qualitative, statistical reporting is not appropriate. Rather, my attempt was to find comment themes and threads running throughout the interviews. Here is what we found. The "community" here is defined as North County, Indiana. While you are reading the following material, you should note that the following paragraphs frequently contain phrases or sentences set off by parentheses. These represent faithful paraphrases of the responses but not verbatim transcripts of responses.

Most Pressing Health Concerns in North County, Indiana

The most frequently mentioned problem was teenage or unplanned pregnancy resulting from peer pressure, poor self-esteem, or poor parenting. North County exhibits the highest rate of teenage pregnancies in Indiana. Pregnant teenagers have unique health problems, and they affect the health of the community because of the psychological, social, and economic cost borne by the woman, her family, and the county's population as a whole.

Access to healthcare services at a reasonable price was the second concern most frequently given. Because of a high proportion of indigent families and low wages, many are not poor enough for Medicaid, but they do not earn enough to purchase health insurance. "Healthcare is generally not available," said one respondent, "if they are not on Medicaid." Another commented that "more services could be provided if healthcare were more accessible to people." A third noted that, because people don't have enough money, they do not have the resources to locate doctors or payment sources.

Substance abuse was a third need identified. The abusive substances of choice in North County were alcohol and marijuana, though respondents felt that LSD and cocaine are abused sometimes. The implications of addiction to alcohol and other drugs for the health of the addict, of his or her family, and of society as a whole are well documented and need not be gone into here.

Other health concerns voiced were sexually transmitted diseases, care of the elderly, domestic violence, and mental health services to nursing homes.

What Is Currently Being Done

At the time, agency representatives felt that little was being done to prevent pregnancies before they occur. Two agencies, though, the North County WIC Program and Planned Parenthood of Northeast/Northwest Indiana, say they are working to alleviate the problems of pregnancy once pregnancy occurs. The WIC program promotes good eating habits during pregnancy and during early childhood and said it was helping find Medicaid funding for pregnant teens and through free pregnancy testing programs. Planned Parenthood of Northeast/Northwest Indiana conducts nutritional counseling, prenatal screening and referrals, community education, and a clinic open one day per week to conduct free screening and exams.

To improve access to adequate medical care at a reasonable cost, North County Memorial Hospital has opened a free clinic for the indigent, and free services are available through Planned Parenthood, and the county also operates a WIC program.

Porter-Cooper Services offers assistance to individuals experiencing stress and respite care for those subject to violence from alcoholism or drug abuse. Also, an alcohol and drug abuse committee has been active in the county within the past year; and the Intervention Youth Program works with addicts through the court system, stressing education, social development, and family dynamics.

How Adequately Current Needs Are Being Met

Welfare department statistics show that North County ranks third lowest of all counties in income per capita and highest in number of case loads per capita. This suggests that current efforts are not enough.

What Should Be Done to Meet These Needs More Adequately

Four approaches are money, education, economic development, and an integrated approach to health problems. First, everyone interviewed cited the need for more money to fund additional staff and more programs, but they further noted that people need to become educated about the consequences of certain health-related behaviors. Second, they argued for a need to convince people of the benefits of changing specific behaviors that lead to substance abuse and unwanted pregnancies. Third, respondents' comments suggest that North County seems to suffer the consequences of a kind of conservative hostility against using services from outside the county, and, at the same time, a reluctance to believe solutions suggested by people within the county. Many felt that people must become more accepting of services from outside the county, because the resources within the county are relatively sparse. The fourth strategy outlined was economic development. Historically, employers in the county have relied on low-skilled workers whom they did not have to pay well. But because healthcare costs are rising faster than wages, there has been an increase in the number of people who cannot afford healthcare. Finally, there was a consensus that favored a coordinated approach to meeting the community's health needs. They noted that the community's approach in the past has been too fragmented by "turf battles."

I noted a rather mixed view of the organization that should head the effort to improve the community's health status. Some respondents indicated that the community hospital should undertake the effort, but others thought it might not be cost-effective to do so. They did not elaborate.

Future Needs

Most respondents were uncomfortable when asked to project what the county may need "down the road." Some see an increase in sexually transmitted diseases, such as AIDS, perhaps an increase in tuberculosis and more cocaine traffic. They did agree that conditions would not change significantly without changes in behavior, education, and more money.

HEALTH PRACTICES AND PATTERNS

As a part of our study of health needs in North County, Indiana, I conducted a telephone survey to find out people's opinions on health practices and opinions about the community's health needs, about their behaviors in seeking medical care, and about their perceptions about healthcare needs in the county. The material in the rest of this chapter is based on telephone interviews with 300 heads of household, randomly selected from North County and the area just outside the county.

Utilization of Hospital Care

An important health indicator is the extent to which people use local hospitals and physicians. It serves as an indicator of how people relate to the medical services delivery system in their community. As a part of our study, we asked people if they had used the services of a hospital, either as an inpatient, outpatient, or emergency. It turned out that this county stood in stark contrast with national trends. We found that 56 percent have used a hospital's emergency room; 82 percent have used inpatient services; and 18 percent have used outpatient services. Nationally, outpatient utilization considerably outstrips inpatient utilization. (See Exhibit 5–3.)

In North County, the opposite is the case; inpatient exceeds outpatient use. I think this shows that, in North County, people relate to their hospitals as people used to in past years. The hospital has remained central to the healthcare system in the county and must play a central role in any efforts to improve the community's health status.

EXHIBIT 5–3
Use of Inpatient, Outpatient, and ER Care
North County, Indiana, 1993

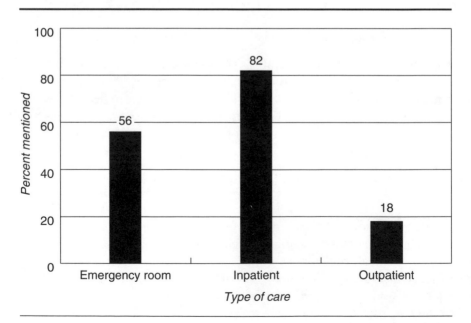

Hospital Patterns

Much attention has been paid to the cost of healthcare. But when people go to the hospital in North County, they want to be taken care of, and they don't consider the cost of medical services. We found that, when people in North County are asked what they think a good hospital means, 46 percent think of good doctors and 10 percent think of good nurses. No one cited inexpensive care as a key attribute of good healthcare. (See Exhibit 5–4).

We asked respondents who had used a hospital how they found out about the hospital they used. When there was no emergency involved, the doctor was the most important factor, followed by word of mouth. People in North County tended to find out about medical services by word of mouth. About 36 percent said they heard about the hospital they use from their physician, and 17 percent found out from friends or relatives. The major reasons cited for choosing a specific hospital were the doctor practicing at the hospital, location close to home, and being taken to a given hospital by an ambulance. (See Exhibit 5–5.)

Physician Patterns

North County is characterized by long-term relationships with physicians. About 86 percent of respondents reported having a regular physician. This figure means that most people have a physician they feel they can rely on

EXHIBIT 5–4
Attributes of a Good Hospital
North County, Indiana, 1993

Preference

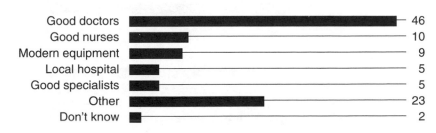

Good doctors	46
Good nurses	10
Modern equipment	9
Local hospital	5
Good specialists	5
Other	23
Don't know	2

Percent response

EXHIBIT 5–5
How People Select Hospitals
North County, Indiana, 1993

Source

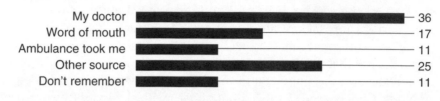

	Percent response
My doctor	36
Word of mouth	17
Ambulance took me	11
Other source	25
Don't remember	11

when they need regular care. Almost all of them have had their physician for at least a year. About 41 percent have had a regular physician for 10 years or more, 67 percent for 5 years or more, 83 percent for 2 years or more, and 93 percent for a year or more. Only 5 percent had been with their physician less than one year. (See Exhibit 5–6.)

EXHIBIT 5–6
Physician Data
North County, Indiana, 1993

Category

Respondents with regular doctor:

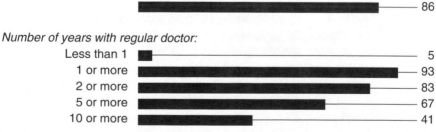

86

Number of years with regular doctor:

	Percent response
Less than 1	5
1 or more	93
2 or more	83
5 or more	67
10 or more	41

How People Select Physicians

People selected their doctors on the basis of word-of-mouth recommendations or because of the location of the doctor. The recommendations of others account for about 54 percent of the decision; location of the doctor accounts for 23 percent; having the doctor practice at the local hospital and the gender of the physician each accounted for 2 percent; insurance requirements for 1 percent; and other reasons for 18 percent. (See Exhibit 5–7.)

EXHIBIT 5–7
Reason for Selecting Physician
North County, Indiana, 1993

Reason cited

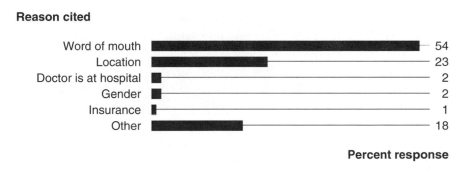

Word of mouth	54
Location	23
Doctor is at hospital	2
Gender	2
Insurance	1
Other	18

Percent response

Access to Medical Services

Not very many people found many problems in finding a physician or specialist. About 84 percent of respondents reported finding their physician very easily, and 12 percent said it had been fairly easy to find a physician. We also asked people whether they had sought the services of a specialist within the past year. Only a very small number of people had looked for a specialist, but couldn't find one.

Perceptions of Health Needs in North County

Community providers identified the need for improved access to lower-priced healthcare and insurance as a priority. Community residents saw this need as well. When asked to identify the community's most pressing health needs, 37 percent cited less costly care, and 13 percent gave the need for more health insurance. (See Exhibit 5–8.)

Of those with insurance, 45 percent participated in group plans, 27 percent in standard plans, and 23 percent in Medicare or Medicaid. Only 3 percent reported being covered by an HMO or PPO, though this percentage may underestimate the penetration of managed care companies, because some of the group plans may be managed care plans.

These results suggest a real insecurity among people in the county, and the insecurity that the data suggest translates into a reluctance among a sizable proportion of respondents to seek medical attention. About 26 percent of respondents reported they had put off seeking medical attention for themselves or others because of lack of money or insurance. This is much higher than other areas we have studied and reflects inadequate healthcare delivery. (See Exhibit 5–9.)

Children are particularly vulnerable. These "outliers" in our society occupy positions that make them less powerful. Yet there was no popular consensus of what they need: 26 percent of those with children and 41 percent of those without children reported having no opinion on the subject. Heading the list for those with children were good emergency care or emergency room, good doctors and pediatricians, and cheaper healthcare.

EXHIBIT 5–8
Key Health Needs
North County, Indiana, 1993

Need cited

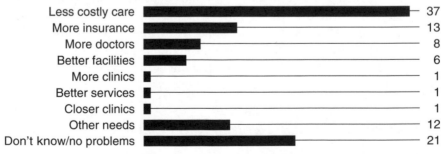

Percent response

EXHIBIT 5–9
Health Insurance Data
North County, Indiana, 1993

Indicator

Respondents who say they are uninsured:

14

Type of insurance of insured respondents:

Group plan	45
Standard plan	27
Medicare/Medicaid	23
HMO/PPO	3
Don't know	2

Respondents who say they are putting off medical attention because of cost:

26

Percent response

But a host of other needs were also mentioned: sex education and teaching about abstinence, therapy, more and better dental care, first-aid training, and others.

At the top of the list for people without children were immunizations, good or better doctors, and sex education and birth control. But other needs cited included these: lower-cost healthcare, better insurance, emergency room care, pediatricians, good clinics, drug education or counseling, and closer doctors. Other items mentioned were immunizations, birth control education, AIDS prevention, "places for recreation," friendly doctors, and eye care. (See Exhibit 5–10.)

Services for the Elderly

The elderly constitute another vulnerable group in society. They are less able to access services on their own. In contrast with public perceptions of children's needs, there was a consensus regarding the needs of the elderly: cheaper healthcare, home healthcare, transportation, and things to do with

EXHIBIT 5–10
Children's Needs
North County, Indiana, 1993

Major need cited

Respondents with children:

Emergency room	14
Good doctor/pediatrician	8
Cheaper care	8
Good care/service	6
Routine care	5
Other responses	33
Don't know	26

Respondents without children:

Immunizations	8
Good/better doctors	5
Sex ed./birth control	4
Low cost/free care	4
Better insurance	3
Closer care/doctors	3
Other	24
None	6
Don't know	41

Percent response

Percentages may not total 100 due to multiple responses.

their peers headed the list. But people who were not care givers of the elderly listed a wide range of needs, including: 24-hour and respite care, emergency care, specialized treatment, better understanding, physical therapy, house calls, and others. Among respondents who were not caring for an elderly friend or relative, there was a much greater range of responses: specialists, better doctors, free nursing homes, faster service, help with activities, preventative care, help with medication, more patience, and others. (See Exhibit 5–11.)

The clearer consensus among people concerning children is especially striking in comparison with the much clearer consensus regarding the

EXHIBIT 5–11
Needs of the Elderly
North County, Indiana, 1993

Need identified

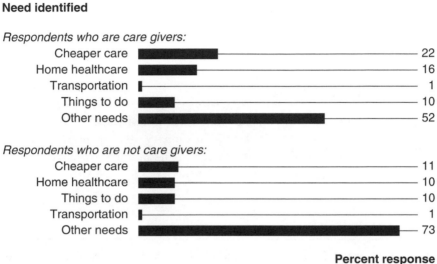

Respondents who are care givers:

Cheaper care	22
Home healthcare	16
Transportation	1
Things to do	10
Other needs	52

Respondents who are not care givers:

Cheaper care	11
Home healthcare	10
Things to do	10
Transportation	1
Other needs	73

Percent response

elderly. Our society has heard a lot about problems of the elderly through newspaper and television coverage and from daily conversation. It could be that for this reason we as a society pay more attention to the elderly than we do our children. After all, we see in the elderly our future; our children are but dim reminders of what we tried to grow away from, and we see them only through the glass darkly. Perhaps we have formed ideas more firmly about the elderly than we do about our children. Perhaps we need to pay more attention to children and their needs, for they will form the society of tomorrow.

Chapter Six

Central California

INTRODUCTION

This chapter presents the results from a community leader survey conducted in Central County, California, in January 1995. It presents a most interesting contrast with the other areas of the country we have studied. Data were collected by phone and from the federal census.

OVERVIEW

In 1990, Central County was home to about 543,477 people, about 1.82 percent of the state's 29,760,021 people. The county accounted for 181,480 households, about 1.7 percent of the state's 10,381,206 households.

Salient Population Characteristics

Exhibit 6–1 displays selected data taken from the 1990 federal census. First, Central County has a somewhat larger household size when compared with the state of California as a whole: 2.92 persons per household, compared with 2.79. Second, in Central County, about 5.8 percent of women over the age of 65 live alone, smaller than the statewide average of 6.0 percent. Third, the median age of residents of Central County, 29.7 years, is 1.7 years lower than the median age of the state, 31.4 years. Fourth, Central County shows a lower educational level than the state as a whole. The percentage of high school dropouts for the county is 3.5 percentage points higher than for the state; the percentage of people enrolled in college is 11.2 percentage points lower than the statewide percentage; and the percentage of the population that has graduated from high school is lower by 8.6 percentage points. Fifth, Central County's employment rate, at 9.7 percent, is considerably higher than the state's unemployment

EXHIBIT 6–1
Population of Central County and State of California Compared

Characteristic	County	State
Mean household size	2.92	2.79
Percent of women over 65, living alone	5.8	6.0
Age distribution:		
Percent under 5	9.6	8.1
Percent under 18	31.5	26.0
Percent 18 to 24	10.0	11.5
Percent 25 to 44	32.6	34.7
Percent 45 to 64	16.2	17.3
Percent 65 or older	1.9	2.3
Percent 80 or older	9.7	10.5
Median age	29.7	31.4
Percent persons aged 16–19, not enrolled in high school, and not graduated	17.7	14.2
Percent persons 18 to 24 enrolled in college	22.1	33.3
Percent high school graduate or higher	67.6	76.2
Percent unemployed	9.7	6.6
Percent foreign born entered 1980–1990	48.6	50.4
Percent foreign born	12.2	21.7
Percent who speak a language other than English and do not speak English "very well"	11.9	16.2
Percent of families for whom poverty status is determined	13.7	9.3
Median household income	$28,634	$35,798

* All population data taken from the United States Census, 1990: *Social and Economic Characteristics*, vol. CP-2-6, Tables 1–3; *General Population Characteristics*, vol. CP-1-6, Tables 1 and 2.

rate of 6.6 percent. Sixth, compared to the state as a whole, Central County has a much smaller percentage of foreign-born, a smaller percentage of people not speaking English well, and a smaller percentage of foreign-born persons who entered between 1985 and 1990. Seventh, the proportion of families below the poverty level is much higher in Central County than it is statewide, 13.7 percent compared with 9.3 percent for the state. Eighth, the county's median household income, $28,634, is only 79.9 percent of the median household income for the state as a whole, $38,798.

Services Available

Central County benefits from a large number and a wide range of social services available to residents through state, county, and private agencies. In contrast with other areas of the country, where people must travel outside the county for services, Central County appears to be rich in the number and variety of service agencies. This analysis, however, can make no assessment of the quality of those services.

Pressing Health Concerns

As does any other area of the country, Central County faces an array of health needs. To establish some priorities about competing health needs, we conducted a special survey of social service agencies serving Central County. As noted earlier, "health" is viewed in this analysis as the physical, emotional, environmental, and psychological well-being of people. The starting point of the study is how the area's health services delivery systems can work most effectively to improve the overall health status of the community.

To identify the most pressing health needs, problems, and issues, we interviewed representatives and organizations active in Central County. Names of agencies and organizations were taken from a 1993 resource directory of community and governmental services. This guide contains listings of over 400 community agencies.

We sampled randomly every 10th agency from this directory. Then we eliminated agencies no longer operating, those located outside of Bakersfield, and those which, during the time allotted to the study, were either unavailable or refused to participate in the study. This produced a final sample of 26 social service and agency representatives interviewed. Most interviews lasted from 5 to 10 minutes. Interviews were conducted between January 17 and March 9, 1995.

Representatives of the following agencies were included in this survey: Central City School District, Central County Health Department, Traffic & Alcohol Awareness Schools of Central County, the National Association for People with Disabilities, Consumer Credit Counseling Service of Central County, California Youth Authority, the chamber of commerce, the American Cancer Society, Protective Services for Children, Employers Training Resource, Maternal Child-Adolescent Support Group, Catholic Social Services, Alano Club, U.S. Probation and Parole, Planned Parenthood of Central California, Friendship House Community Center,

Lutheran Social Services of Southern California, Lupus Support Group, Hearts Connection Family Resource/Support Center, California Retired Teachers' Association, Aware, Inc., Delano Ministerial Association, Centre for Neuro Skills, Arthritis Association of Central County, Pacific Medical Service, and Central County coroner and public administrator.

This chapter frequently contains quoted passages. The reader should note these represent accurate paraphrases of respondents' remarks, not actual quotations, which have been altered to protect the confidentiality of the respondent. The reader should also remember that the comments reflect perceptions only. We have made no attempt to verify the truth of individual responses, nor could we have done so.

The Most Pressing Health Need

The interview began by pointing out that the purpose of our study was to "gain your perspective concerning the most important health issues, problems, or concerns in Central County." After collecting some background information, we asked respondents the following question: "We're interested in your perspective as a person who is active in the affairs of your county, and we are looking at health in a very broad context, one that incorporates environmental, emotional, and psychological well-being in addition to the absence of disease. From this perspective, then, what would you say is the most pressing health problem, issue, or concern in Central County right now?" The first response that came to mind was written down.

Seven respondents gave as most important a very complex group of needs related to lack of healthcare services for the disadvantaged, including the high cost of medical treatment and insurance and poor access to healthcare. The major factor limiting access is that only one hospital in the county will treat low-income patients on a regular basis. Many respondents noted a strong reluctance among the other hospitals to focus on treating those who either pay their own bills or have private medical insurance. The rest are left to Central Medical Center. Because many low-income people cannot afford health insurance, or are not eligible for public assistance, they often are denied access to the medical service delivery systems. Further, others who do not have easy access to transportation or an understanding of how or where to look may be medically "disenfranchised" as well.

One respondent said that "the biggest problem we have is healthcare for the migrant worker. This becomes a problem because there is only one clinic and one hospital that will treat them. Healthcare for them is generally not available." Another agreed that "the resources available for the disadvantaged are few. The number of available programs and services for the disadvantaged are so limited that they don't know where to turn for healthcare." A third: "The primary need is the socioeconomic concerns of unemployment. This is related to substance abuse and teen pregnancy, and results in high school dropouts, unemployment, family and domestic violence, and problems in schools because kids don't get identification early and the help they need." A fourth: "The most pressing issue is the high cost of medical treatment and insurance. It denies assess to those who can't afford it and means no treatment for those people." A fifth: "The biggest problem is access to healthcare in general. We have a group with no insurance that doesn't get any healthcare. As a result, they spread illnesses and disease to the rest of us. It also produces absenteeism and keeps kids out of school." A sixth noted that the most pressing need is "the lack of availability of low-cost health insurance for people of low income. They can't find a doctor that takes MediCal." And a seventh: "There's lots of no health insurance. A lot of our economy is agricultural. Most agricultural labor is seasonal. Seasonal work results in children without immunization, and children can only get taken care of in the county hospital. As a result, we have a higher incidence of disease."

Related to the above needs are infant mortality, prenatal care, and proper medical care for children, which were discussed slightly by five respondents A major need is to increase the proportion of children who are immunized. Lack of immunizations put the community at risk because of the too-rapid spread of infectious diseases. Needed also was better prenatal care, the lack of which leads to increased rate of disability, creates increased need for special education, jeopardizes the overall quality of care in the community, and places an insupportably high burden on the healthcare system. Finally, respondents highlighted a lack of understanding among parents concerning proper medical treatment for children. Further, there is a lack of transportation for families to regularly take children to doctors.

Here are some representative quotes. (1) "Infant mortality and prenatal care are high in our region. This has definite fiscal implications. Cost is tied to their care, and it affects the health population later in life. It produces more people with disabilities, increases the number of kids in special education, and damages the quality of life in our community." (2) "There's a need for better immunization and better medical care for children. There is just a large number of women who don't get their kids treated when they need it. There is little transportation for families that don't have cars, and there is a general lack of knowledge on the part of parents so that they know how to take care of their children." (3) "The biggest problem is lack of children's services. Healthcare for kids, such as immunization, gets neglected because of economics." (4) "The immunization rate for children under two years old is the lowest in the state. They spread measles, chicken pox, and other kinds of things." (5) "There are not enough services for pregnant women. So many come with no money and high risks."

Four other needs—mental health, violence, teen pregnancy, and substance abuse—flow directly from these problems. Mental health problems occur when "there are not enough services for middle-income people who have too much money to qualify for MediCal. Counseling fees are at least $45 per hour and rise steeply with income." Further, "We have a lot of mental health problems. People are treated and released to homes where there are serious mental health problems, and resources are not sufficient to meet the problem." The problem of violence is embodied in "drive-by shootings, youth killings, and domestic violence, and it is harder to get emergency personnel and health workers into the homes because of the perceived danger." Another respondent elaborated: "Antisocial behavior is our biggest problem. Parents lack the skills to teach appropriate skills, and as a result we have a higher rate of violence and aggressive behavior." Teen pregnancy "burdens the welfare system, damages social mores, and places a burden on our healthcare system." "There's just a lot of it," noted another; "we're first or second in the state in terms of teen pregnancies." A man said, "substance abuse is a serious problem, with effects which carry over into the family." He might have noted that they contribute to all these other problems as well as flow from them.

Five respondents singled out valley fever, a very dangerous illness resulting from a fungus in the soil, which leads to other illnesses, such as meningitis. Valley fever affects everyone and has very serious implications, because there is no known cure. "It used to be quite isolated. It can be fatal, and it takes everyone out of work. It keeps them in the hospital for the long-term."

Other problems noted were a lack of skilled medical specialists in the area, a lack of financial security for retired teachers, a need for better geriatric services in a growing older population, and AIDS.

Current Actions Being Taken to Meet the Needs

Next we asked respondents to discuss current efforts to meet these needs and to evaluate how well the needs were being met. There appear to be some initiatives to improve the quality of services for the indigent and disadvantaged and children. One respondent referred to "some health clinics," another to the fact that "the county is doing what it can." The health department apparently is working to place public health nurses in high-risk neighborhoods, and it has distributed posters and leaflets door to door. Further, there have been attempts to increase the proportion of infants who have been immunized. However, one respondent's assessment, "talk, not much else," apparently summarizes the opinions of most respondents. Echoing these opinions are those discussing efforts to deal with other health problems. To address the lack of mental health services, little has been done. To diminish the incidence of teen pregnancy, respondents saw the need for new or better parenting classes for parents and sex education courses for teens, as well as low-cost clinics for pregnant or at-risk teens. There apparently has been some effort on the part of the health department to form a coalition to discuss how to deal with increased violence, and some effort on the part of the schools to teach parenting and social skills. To combat valley fever, respondents referred to studies that have been undertaken, a task force to discuss how to deal with the problem, and efforts to develop a vaccine.

Actions Needed to Successfully Address the Issues

To address other issues than valley fever, respondents stressed three factors: more money, working together better, and a stronger, more proactive approach. There certainly was no disagreement that more money would help. "Not much better can be done without more money," said one respondent. However, stronger collaboration was noted by many: "We need an active children's network, to address healthcare issues for children," said one respondent. Another added that efforts have been minimal; "agencies have to work together to get organized."

One respondent stressed the need for more grassroots lobbying and legislative efforts. With regard to valley fever, most respondents professed ignorance of what strategies should be employed.

Role of the Community Hospital

There is a clear sense that, to address most problems, close collaboration by a number of different agencies should be employed. In contrast to most areas we have studied, local hospitals are not seen as primary participants in working with community agencies. Rather, comments reflect a view that hospitals primarily provide medical services and are not needed to get involved in working with community agencies.

Further, I sensed a high level of suspicion and cynicism concerning the purposes and uses of the research conducted. Taken together, these two conclusions suggest that extra efforts may be required to work effectively with local agencies, especially if they view the actions of others outside their own agencies as at best suspicious.

The Extent to Which Hospitals Are Meeting Their Communities' Pressing Health Needs

To gauge respondents' opinions of how well the local hospitals are doing to meet the overall health needs of the community, respondents were asked the following: "Next, I'd like to get some idea of how well you think local hospitals are doing to meet Central County's health needs. I am going to give you each hospital by name, and after I do, please tell me, if you were to grade the hospital, like in school, where A is excellent and F is failing, what grade you would give it."

Many respondents did not feel qualified to evaluate the local hospitals. A characteristic response was the following: "We don't do much with the local hospitals. From what I have heard, they're all pretty good. There aren't any I wouldn't go to." However, many did offer opinions of the various hospitals, and each hospital is discussed in turn. Grade points for each hospital are shown in Exhibit 6–2; explanations for giving selected grades are given in the next section.

Hospital Grades

Memorial Hospital received a "grade point average" of 3.43, a normal grade for a hospital. It received generally high marks for being community-minded and having an excellent cardiac unit, but is graded down by some for not taking low-income patients. (See Exhibit 6–2.)

Central City's grade point average, 3.41, is quite acceptable. It gets good marks for its high overall level of care and involvement in the community. However, some respondents have commented on delays in admitting and emergency room, for a lack of responsiveness to patients, and some downgraded the hospital for not treating low-income patients.

Grades for Central County Medical Center were somewhat lower than most hospitals, but fairly good for a public hospital. The hospital gets downgraded because it is viewed as having an unsavory and unsafe atmosphere. It also gets low marks for being understaffed, which often results in long waits. However, many respondents give it higher grades for

EXHIBIT 6–2
Grades for Area Hospitals
Central California, 1995

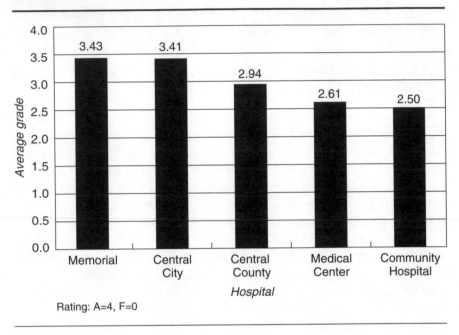

Rating: A=4, F=0

taking low-income patients; it is the only area provider, apparently, which does so on a regular basis.

At 2.50, grades for Community Hospital are below average. The hospital gets good marks for having a good cardiac unit, but the physical plant appears to be a bit old and needs to be improved. Further, respondents downgraded the hospital because it needs to do a better job of serving the community.

Explanations for Grades and What Each Hospital Needs to Do Better

Memorial Hospital (14 graders, GPA=3.43)

- A: "They have an exceptional cardiac unit with state of the art equipment."
- A: "A good hospital, but not very community-oriented."

- A: "A top hospital. They continually upgrade their services and keep the community aware of their efforts."
- A: "Facilities are great, personnel are well trained, and they give a good deal of confidence."
- A: "Great—they have reached out in the community and networked."
- A: "It is doing a good job. All my contacts have been positive."
- A: "It has a neonatal intensive care unit. Birth defect and premature babies are well cared for there."
- A: "It is a good hospital, especially its emergency room."
- B: "Doesn't deal with Medicaid or MediCal. It does fine with private payers, and it is respected in the community. It works with community agencies more than before."
- B: "They have done an adequate job. They have a lot of new construction, but they don't get involved with low-income patients."
- B: "There is a serious lack of nurses. They need to get more nurses."
- C: "They need more nurses and to be more responsive to patients. We hear stories about people being ignored even when pushing their buttons."
- C: "They are good at what they do, but they don't treat low-income patients."
- D: "They need to make more resources available to the community."

Central County (18 graders; GPA=2.94)

- A: "They are the only hospital that treats low-income patients. It has a reputation for long waits and being unsafe. It has the best trauma unit, and does the best it can."
- A: "It is primarily for indigent and MediCal patients. They are making some changes with WIC patients. But there are long waits for individuals, and the staff is not as sensitive to people as it should be. But they do take on everyone."
- A: "For what they have, they are excellent."
- A: "They have a brand new emergency room."
- A: "All the hospitals are great."
- B: "For a county facility it has a pretty good reputation. It takes low-income people. But it has long waiting times to get in. It's a teaching hospital and gives good training over there."
- B: "Its emergency room is very slow. People are just left for hours and people are working their butts off there."

- B: "For its purpose it does well. It focuses on people with MediCal or Medicaid insurance. People wait a long time in the emergency room."
- B: "The majority of people are Medicare or MediCal. I try to get out of there as soon as possible."
- B: "The ER deserved an A, and they have the best trauma unit and a helicopter. The rest of it gets a B/B+.
- B: "They're good at what they do. They have begun to streamline their system to speed things up. They will have a new facility with more space, and people will flow faster."
- B: "There is a problem with long waits."
- B: "It is available to everyone, on a 24-hour basis. It needs increased funding to improve its services."
- C: "They are overwhelmed with what they have to deal with as a county facility."
- C: "Make services more convenient so they can serve more people in a day."
- C: "A county hospital. I don't know if they have funding problems or what, but it is just not well staffed. They need more staff."
- C: "It needs more funding for more staff."
- D: "This is the worst—overpopulated. People wait for hours if they are not critically hurt."

Community Hospital (17 graders; GPA=2.50)

- A: "It keeps up to date and has a well-trained staff."
- A: "Its cardiac unit is exceptional; staffed 24 hours."
- B: "Not from experience; just from what I've heard."
- B: "It has a very good heart center. It does excellent seminars in the community."
- B: "It is a good hospital, but the personnel are cold and seem to be preoccupied."
- B: "I don't have a specific reason."
- B: "No reason I know of."
- B: "They do a good job of giving people good care."
- B: "They don't have the community access that the other hospitals have."
- B: "The emergency room is fine. I don't know what it would take to get an A."

- B: "It is not well kept up. It needs to invest some resources on expanding."
- B: "It has made big improvements by opening up a maternity wing."
- B: "It needs to broaden its emergency room services and expedite things for those who need help. It is very slow."
- B: "It needs more money for more staff."
- B: "It is very old and needs to be updated."
- C: "The staff is good at what it does, but it doesn't treat low-income people."
- D: "It doesn't serve the community very well. It needs to do more community outreach."

Central City (18 graders; GPA=3.41)

- A: "It gives good care to insured people. It is treating more Medi-Cal people now, though."
- A: "It has an excellent cancer treatment center, and a new hospital near me."
- A: "The nurses are fine."
- A: "It has an outreach program in the southeast part of town. The hospital is involved in the community and encourages its employees to do so as well."
- A: "It has good facilities, including excellent intensive care and cardiac units, and the staff is very professional. There aren't as many staff in the ER compared with the other hospitals, but they respond well."
- A: "It is very involved in the community."
- A: No reason given.
- B: "They donate funds for community organizations, gifts, and clothes, etc. They need to hire or have staff familiar with the Afro-American community."
- B: "They expanded into the community, and do an excellent of serving the whole community. But they don't treat MediCal patients."
- B: "They need to broaden their emergency room services and speed up services."
- B: "It is a good hospital, but the waits are too long."
- B: "Their admitting is slow, but they give excellent care."

- B: "They need to improve their outreach into the community and bring down costs."
- C: "It is a religious hospital, with two centers for accessibility. I don't know much about it."
- C: "They need more nurses, or to be more responsive to patients. I hear stories about people being left alone even when pushing their buttons. They just don't respond for some reason."
- C: "It is good at what it does, but it doesn't treat low-income people."

CONCLUSIONS FROM THE CENTRAL COUNTY STUDY

First, respondents see not enough being done to offer better access to the medical services delivery system by unemployed, disadvantaged, and low-income residents of Central County. The lack of services results in insufficient immunizations, and in domestic violence, teenage pregnancy, substance abuse, and a host of related medical problems.

Second, the survey showed a need for better prenatal, neonatal, and other services for children and their parents. Because of lack of knowledge, social skills, and income, not enough children are immunized, and an undesirable high rate of children with disabilities and poor healthcare will grow up to be unhealthy adults who place a serious drain on the local healthcare system.

Third, there is widespread agreement of a need for a cure for valley fever. Because it affects everyone in the county, current efforts to find a cure should be continued.

I was quite struck by the high level of cynicism and suspicion surrounding my efforts to interview people. The proportion of potential respondents who declined to be interviewed, and who finally consented to participate only after extensive questioning, was substantially higher than in any other area we have studied. Seldom was my effort accepted at face value. In almost every case, respondents wondered who I was, why I was conducting the research, and how it would be used. I believe this reflects a troubling level of "turfism," a level that may jeopardize efforts to reach out to community agencies in an honest and straightforward way.

I was also impressed by the lack of knowledge of the activities of the hospitals in Central County. Respondents did not know very much about the hospitals or had only a passing familiarity with them. Responses to the question of what organizations should be responsible for addressing the health needs of the area seldom included any of the local providers. I believe that respondents see hospitals only as providers of medical services, not as active community organizations. If the hospitals in Central County wish to take their place as a valued community organization, they are going to have to work harder to reach out to the entire community.

I was struck, too, by respondents' criticism of Central County Medical Center as being too crowded and slow. Apparently, the county facility is overcrowded because the other hospitals are either reluctant to treat low-income patients, or treat only a few of them. Central County Medical Center then becomes a provider of last resort.

Apparently there have been efforts to reach out to the community. However, hospitals should work to expand their efforts to embrace the community and to foster close working relationships, which will help them build stronger bridges to community organizations. Hospitals may wish to accomplish this through beefing up their educational programs: to increase the public understanding of disease, to improve the social skills of teens and young adults, and to improve the parenting skills of young parents.

Finally, we agree with the respondent who favored a three-pronged approach to solving problems: a proactive approach, better collaboration, and more resources.

Chapter Seven

Inner City, Ohio, 1992

INTRODUCTION

This study differs from our assessments in that it was carried out by the county health board. I assisted with the overall effort, specifically with evaluating the research and analysis. A community planning agency assisted the board with research design, questionnaire development, and data analysis. The Center for Urban Poverty and Social Change, affiliated with a major university in the city, provided an extended analysis of census data for the city.

BACKGROUND AND PURPOSE

The Board of Health became the official health agency for Inner City, Ohio, in April of 1990. The first year of operation over the city made clear to the board that it needed a clearer understanding of the community's health concerns and beliefs to enable the board to provide the programs and other activities that would meet the needs of the community. According to the study report:

> The study was designed to capture present conditions affecting public health, the ability of residents to access health services, and their perceptions of environmental and public health concerns; such a comprehensive effort provided the Board with a knowledge-base to be utilized in its long-range plan for the community.

Once the research was completed, an "implementation" committee was formed to review the study findings and develop recommendations for the Board of Health to consider. The recommendations will enable the Board of Health to utilize its own resources as well as to mobilize other providers to provide optimal health services to the community.

METHODOLOGY

The study relied on a mix of survey techniques. First, a survey of 206 households collected information on the perceived healthcare needs of residents. Households were randomly selected, using 1990 U.S. census data to construct a block-level profile of the community. Specific addresses were selected from a directory by means of a fixed interval selection procedure. This resulted in a geographic distribution of households throughout the city and a representative sample of the population in terms of key sociodemographic variables. To ensure that the senior population was represented, seniors were selected from clients of a local senior center. An 18-page data collection instrument was developed to gather information on household characteristics, health status, and healthcare utilization patterns of residents, plus perceptions of selected environmental/public health issues. The survey included both structured and open-ended questions. Interviewers were hired and trained in interviewing techniques and in the use of the questionnaire. Data were collected via door-to-door interviews.

Second, interviews with representatives of 56 health and social service provider agencies obtained information on environmental and public health issues affecting community residents. Representatives of social service agencies serving the community were identified by the staff of the board. These included representatives of city government, local hospitals, private practices, community agencies, churches, and civic agencies. Two survey instruments elicited information on their perceptions and experiences regarding important environmental or public health issues. This format included structured as well as open-ended questions.

Third, 321 students from two community schools were surveyed to obtain information on the healthcare issues affecting adolescents. Students for the sample were selected randomly from health classes in grades 6–12. Students completed a self-administered questionnaire, consisting of a subset of questions from the household survey and focusing on the health status of the students and recent use of medical services.

Finally, analysis of census data provided a "snapshot" of the sociodemographic structure of the community.

RESEARCH QUESTIONS

The research covered the following topics: the characteristics of the city's population; the current health status of the city; the healthcare utilization patterns of the city; the perceived barriers to the healthcare delivery system; the environmental problems residents perceive as important; the public health problems residents perceive as important; and the perception of health needs of city residents by service providers.

Socioeconomic Trends, 1980–1990

The analysis of socioeconomic data for the city, compared with the county, showed that poverty, and factors associated with it, was a particular problem in Inner City, Ohio. (See Exhibit 7–1.)

EXHIBIT 7–1
Poverty and Welfare Dependency, 1990

Indicator	City	County
AFDC recipients per 1,000 population	102.0	38.9
General assistance per 1,000 population	75.1	28.4
Food stamp per 1,000 population	365.0	141.0
Medicaid recipients per 1,000 population	42.7	22.4
Poverty per 1,000 population	33.2	14.9

Analysis of data from the U.S. census shows that the decade of the 1980s brought increasing hardships to the city's population. A review of quality of life indicators shows that the city became poorer as more residents became dependent on government for income maintenance and health insurance. Although the trend toward increased poverty and public sector dependence has occurred in the county as a whole, it had increased in the city at a much faster rate. For example, since 1980 the rate for assistance for Families with Dependent Children recipients has increased 67 percent in the city, compared with 58 percent for the county; the general assistance rate has risen in the city by 270 percent compared to 209 for the county; the food stamp rate has increased in the city by 345 percent, compared with 229 percent in the county; the poverty rate for the city has increased by 49 percent in the community, compared with 32 percent in the county; and the Medicaid (nonassistance) rate for the city has climbed 91 percent over the decade, compared with 53 percent in the county.

Further analysis of census data also showed a clear shift toward a more racially imbalanced population. The proportion of blacks increased from 87 to 94 percent, while the number of whites decreased from 12 to 5 percent. The proportion of Hispanics and other ethnic or racial groups remained relatively constant at 1.0 to 1.3 percent throughout the decade.

Other aspects of the city's population shifted as well. The proportion of the nonwhite older adult population increased from 10.7 to 16.6 percent; the population of whites aged 55 or over increased from 52 to 54 percent; the proportion of nonwhite children, those under the age of 15, decreased from 26 to 25 percent, but the proportion of white children under the age of 5 decreased by 3 percentage points to 4 percent.

THE HOUSEHOLD SURVEY

Of 206 respondents, 64 percent were women. Over 91 percent were black, and 71 percent were high school graduates or higher. Two-thirds were single. About 28 percent, the largest group of single respondents, were those who have been estranged, separated, or divorced from their spouses. About 51 percent were employed at the time of the survey, and about 52 percent had lived in their current homes for more than five years. The study found no clear differences between men and women, except that males were more likely to be living alone and more likely to be employed.

For purposes of presentation, households were categorized in two ways, first by income and household size, and then by household composition. By income, those at or below the poverty level, as defined by the U.S. Department of Health and Human Services' poverty income guidelines, were defined as very low income; those between the poverty level and 150 percent of the poverty level were defined as low income; and those more than 150 percent of the poverty level were defined as moderate income. About 22 percent were considered very low income, 19 percent were low income, and 59 percent were moderate income. Classified by household composition, those with one adult parent with children younger than 18 years were classified as single parent; households headed by two or more adults with children under the age of 18 years were defined as adults with children; and those headed by a senior, over the age of 60 years, with or without children under the age of 18, were defined as senior-headed. About 13 percent were single parent households, 20 percent were adult with children households, 32 percent were adult-only households, and 35 percent were senior-headed households. Finally, analysis of the respondents showed that 36 percent of households have children; 36 percent have seniors; 43 percent are single-headed households; and 46 percent are female-headed households.

Curiously, the research found a relatively high proportion of families covered by health insurance. According to the report, 94 percent are covered by health insurance, 51 percent by employer-paid, 15 percent by Medicare, 9 percent by Medicaid, 3 percent by self-pay, 2 percent by general assistance, and 11 percent by a combination of coverages. (See Exhibits 7–2 and 7–3.)

HEALTH STATUS INDICATORS

Illnesses and Conditions among Children

Children under the age of 18 were present in 75 of the sample's households. These households contained 142 children, an average of 1.89 children per household. In almost every case, parents reported that their children were in good or excellent health. However, of the children in the sample, 20 percent reported having illnesses that could be classified as serious health problems—mostly asthma, nutritional anemia, sickle cell anemia, lead poisoning, or some sort of disability. Nearly 49 percent of students reported missing school during the past four to six weeks due to illness or injury. (See Exhibit 7–4.)

Cardiovascular Disease in Adults

Health problems and illnesses related to cardiovascular disease were the most commonly reported conditions among adults. Overall, 35 percent of adults reported having seen a physician for high blood pressure, but over 60 percent of households headed by seniors had one or more adults reporting they were currently being treated for high blood pressure. (See Exhibit 7–5.)

Diabetes in Adults

Diabetes was reported among adults in 12 percent of all households. Again, the majority of cases were found in senior-headed households, 27 percent of which reported having one or more adults with diabetes.

EXHIBIT 7–2
Characteristics of Respondents
Inner City, Ohio, 1992

Characteristic

Respondents who are head of household:
— 80

Respondents who are black:
— 91

Respondents who are female:
— 64

Marital status:
Single/not married — 18
Married/cohabitating — 33
Divorced/separated/estranged — 28
Widowed — 21

Respondents who are employed:
— 51

Education:
Not high school grad. — 29
High school graduate — 34
Some college — 20
College graduate — 17

Mean age of respondents:
— 49.6*

Respondents who have resided in the city…
Less than 1 year — 10
1 to 1.9 years — 20
2 to 4.9 years — 18
More than 4.9 years — 52

Percent response

*Not a percentage.

EXHIBIT 7–3
Additional Characteristics of Respondents
Inner City, Ohio, 1992

Characteristic

Income:

Very low	22
Low	19
Moderate	59

Mean household size:

2.29*

Respondents who own homes:

37

Households:

With children	36
With seniors	36
Single person	43
Female-headed	46

Age:

0 to 4 years old	10
5 to 17 years old	21
18 to 59 years old	52
More than 59 years old	17

Children present:

Single parent	13
Adults with children	20
Adults only	32
Senior-headed	35

Percent response

*Not a percentage.

EXHIBIT 7–4
Health Insurance Data
Inner City, Ohio, 1992

Characteristic

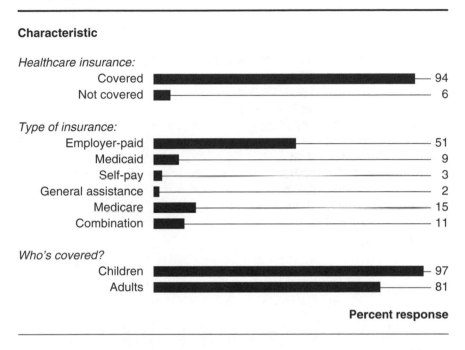

Healthcare insurance:
Covered — 94
Not covered — 6

Type of insurance:
Employer-paid — 51
Medicaid — 9
Self-pay — 3
General assistance — 2
Medicare — 15
Combination — 11

Who's covered?
Children — 97
Adults — 81

Percent response

Heart Attacks and Strokes among Adults

Further, of the households headed by seniors, 11 percent reported having at least one adult who had suffered a heart attack, and 11 percent reported having one adult who had suffered a stroke.

Alcohol and Drug Abuse among Adults

About 8 percent of respondents indicated they or someone in their household had an alcohol or drug problem, mostly related to alcohol. About 38 percent of these also said that the abuser had been in treatment within the past 12 months, another 50 percent had received treatment more than 12 months ago, and the remaining 12 percent reported never having been treated.

EXHIBIT 7–5
Illnesses Reported among Young Adults
Inner City, Ohio, 1992

Condition reported

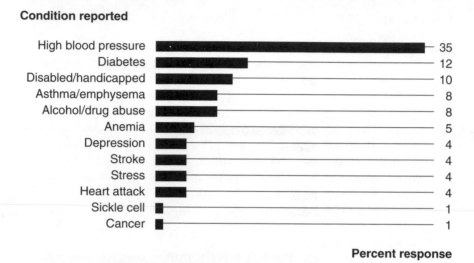

High blood pressure	35
Diabetes	12
Disabled/handicapped	10
Asthma/emphysema	8
Alcohol/drug abuse	8
Anemia	5
Depression	4
Stroke	4
Stress	4
Heart attack	4
Sickle cell	1
Cancer	1

Percent response

ACCESS TO HEALTHCARE RESOURCES

Childhood Immunization

To assess the immunization of preschoolers, adults were asked to produce a written immunization record for their children. Of 36 households with preschoolers, 24 were able to produce written immunization records on 31 children. Twenty-eight of these records were judged accurate on their face. Based on analysis of these 28 records, 35 percent of children had all their required DTP shots, 42 percent had all their recommended OPV doses, and 85 percent had received their first MMR shots. Only 42 percent of mothers had ever consulted with a doctor or taken their children for shots.

Use of Health Resources

All respondents in households with children reported having a "regular" source of medical care, primarily hospital clinics, private physicians, or other health centers or clinics. Only 5 percent reported a hospital emergency room or urgent care center as their children's primary source of care. About 76 percent of all households with children reported visiting a doctor within the past 12 months. Preschoolers were more likely than school-age children to have been seen by a doctor within the past 12 months. (See Exhibit 7–6.)

Low Birth-Weight Babies, Premature Births, and Teen Births

To determine the prevalence of low birth-weight and premature deliveries among the sample, the researchers asked female respondents how many babies they had delivered within the past five years. Over this period, 27 women reported 34 live births, 2.9 percent of the babies were born premature, and 5.9 percent were low birth weight.

About 41 percent of women between the ages of 19 and 40 gave birth to their first child as a teenager, accounting for 20.5 percent of all births for this age cohort, assuming only one teenage birth per woman. Teenagers who are parents suffer a higher rate of poverty than women who are older when they have children. More women who gave birth as a teen now live

EXHIBIT 7–6
Children's Use of Services
Inner City, Ohio, 1992

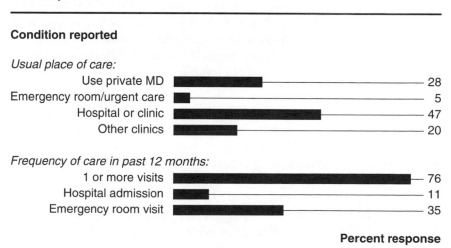

Condition reported

Usual place of care:

Use private MD	28
Emergency room/urgent care	5
Hospital or clinic	47
Other clinics	20

Frequency of care in past 12 months:

1 or more visits	76
Hospital admission	11
Emergency room visit	35

Percent response

in poverty than those women who were not teenage mothers. Teen mothers are more likely than others to be receiving AFDC or general assistance and less likely than others to live in households benefiting from income from a job. Further, they give birth to more children; and they are less likely to be employed, compared to 61 percent of their counterparts.

Adults' Use of Health Resources

About 13 percent of adults reported no regular source of medical care. About 44 percent identified a hospital clinic as the respondent's source of regular care, and 29 percent gave a physician. Only 1 percent gave a hospital emergency room or urgent care center. In 78 percent of the households surveyed, one or more adults had not had any medical visit within the past 12 months; 25 percent of households reported at least one adult hospital admission in the past 12 months by one or more adults; and 31 percent of households reported one or more adults going to a hospital emergency room within the past 12 months. (See Exhibit 7–7.)

Barriers Blocking Access to Healthcare

Researchers asked respondents to identify factors that prevented or made difficult access to healthcare in the area. The three factors mentioned most often were long waits at the office, long waits to get an appointment, poor transportation, and inadequate insurance. Lost pay from work, poor continuity of care, inconvenient hours, lack of knowing "where to go," lack of child care, no phone, and discrimination were also mentioned. These results document the problems low-income families experience in gaining access to the healthcare system. (See Exhibit 7–8.)

Dental Care

One quarter of children of school age in the sample had no regular dentist; 47 percent of adults and 55 percent of all seniors had no dentist. Of children of school age, 42 percent had not visited a dentist within the past year. Of adults, 29 percent had not visited a dentist within the past three years, and an additional 31 percent had not been to a dentist in over three years. Of seniors, 36 percent had not been to a dentist in the past one to three years, and another 33 percent had not been to a dentist in over three years.

EXHIBIT 7–7
Adults' Use of Services
Inner City, Ohio, 1992

Condition reported

Usual place of care:

Use private MD	29
Emergency room/urgent care	1
Hospital or clinic	44
Other clinics	12
None	13

Frequency of care in past 12 months:

1 or more visits	22
Hospital admission	25
Emergency room visit	31

Percent response

EXHIBIT 7–8
Barriers to Medical Care
Inner City, Ohio, 1992

Condition reported

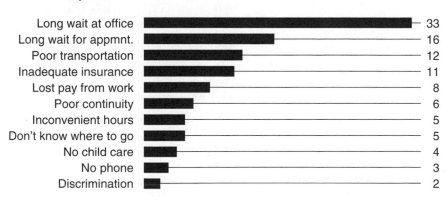

Long wait at office	33
Long wait for appmnt.	16
Poor transportation	12
Inadequate insurance	11
Lost pay from work	8
Poor continuity	6
Inconvenient hours	5
Don't know where to go	5
No child care	4
No phone	3
Discrimination	2

Percent response

To determine the types of environmental and public health problems that concern Inner City, respondents were presented with a list of 13 public health and environmental issues. They were asked to indicate whether they felt each issue was a problem in their city. Of environmental issues, vacant lots and buildings were identified by 68 percent, and 67 percent selected unclean food establishments as the most pressing environmental issue. Of public health issues, teenage pregnancy was chosen by 67 percent, and healthcare for seniors and infant mortality by 40 percent each. Researchers then asked respondents to give a priority to health problems by citing those problems they see as most important. Heading this condensed list of environmental problems were vacant lots and buildings at 25 percent, followed by unsanitary food establishments at 20 percent. Heading the condensed list of public health problems was teenage pregnancy, chosen as most important by 39 percent; followed by infant mortality, chosen as most important by 15 percent; and healthcare for seniors by 14 percent. (See Exhibit 7–9.)

PROVIDER SURVEY

Researchers surveyed 56 agencies providing service to the city to determine their perceptions concerning important environmental and public health issues facing city residents. Fifteen agencies were asked about environmental issues; 41 agencies were asked about public health issues. Researchers used the same list that was presented to household respondents. Almost three-quarters of provider representatives identified vacant lots and derelict buildings as key. Following in importance were unsanitary yards and neighborhoods, rat infestation, and lead poisoning. The following three issues were most frequently identified as key public health issues: HIV, AIDS, and other sexually transmited diseases, identified by 54 percent; pregnancy prevention by 46 percent; and infant mortality by 34 percent. Exhibit 7–10 displays these percentages.

CONCLUSIONS AND IMPLICATIONS

It was clear from the study that the socioeconomic position of people relative to the medical service delivery system was greatly affected by their abilities to gain access to medical care. Disadvantaged people are more

EXHIBIT 7–9
Public Concerns
Inner City, Ohio, 1992

Condition reported

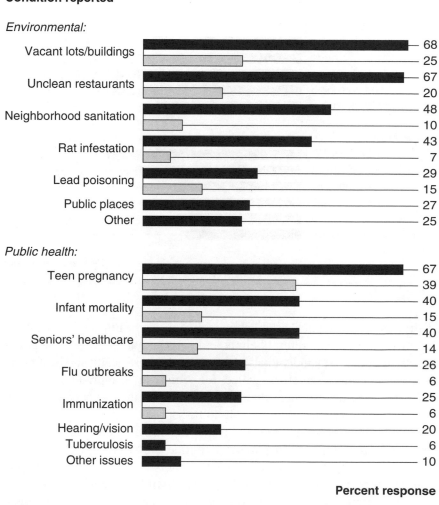

Environmental:

Vacant lots/buildings	68 / 25
Unclean restaurants	67 / 20
Neighborhood sanitation	48 / 10
Rat infestation	43 / 7
Lead poisoning	29 / 15
Public places	27
Other	25

Public health:

Teen pregnancy	67 / 39
Infant mortality	40 / 15
Seniors' healthcare	40 / 14
Flu outbreaks	26 / 6
Immunization	25 / 6
Hearing/vision	20
Tuberculosis	6
Other issues	10

Percent response

■ A problem   ▨ Most important

EXHIBIT 7–10
Providers' Immediate Concerns
Inner City, Ohio, 1992

Concern

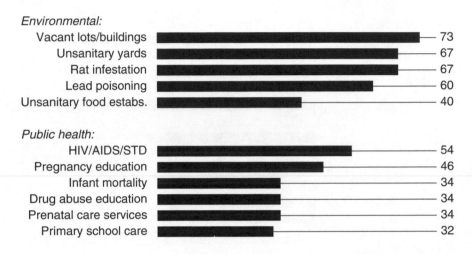

Environmental:
Vacant lots/buildings	73
Unsanitary yards	67
Rat infestation	67
Lead poisoning	60
Unsanitary food estabs.	40

Public health:
HIV/AIDS/STD	54
Pregnancy education	46
Infant mortality	34
Drug abuse education	34
Prenatal care services	34
Primary school care	32

Percent response

distrustful of the medical establishment and utilize health services less frequently. In addition, cultural beliefs and practices among minority populations affect the way individuals and families address health and healthcare issues. The study, therefore, called for "innovative approaches" to the delivery of medical services that take into account the socioeconomic and cultural characteristics of the people to be served.

Beyond this, the study made the following six recommendations. First, because many children do not have routine contacts with the medical system, the study recommended that programs be developed to provide annual checkups for minority children as possible. Second, because the verifiable immunization coverage for preschoolers was poor, efforts need to be made to immunize as many of these children. Third, the study found a higher than expected rate of asthma among children and recommended that efforts be made to target asthma among children. Fourth, because teenage pregnancy was identified as a key health problem, and because the study found a higher than expected rate of teenage pregnancy, the study recommended that programs be developed to reduce the rate of teenage pregnancy. Fifth, the study found a lower than desired utilization rate of prenatal services by pregnant women and recommended that prenatal services be expanded and promoted in the city. Sixth, the study determined that residents were not getting adequate dental care, because they either felt they didn't need it or couldn't afford to pay. The study, therefore, recommended that educational efforts be made to inform residents of the need for dental care and to make it accessible to them.

Chapter Eight

Current Models of Community Health Needs Assessment

INTRODUCTION

Chapter One presented the basic steps through which your hospital can work in collaboration with your community to assess the health of your community and implement plans for change. The process I outlined had 10 steps, organized into three phases. The first phase I called the *planning* phase, and it consisted of the first step: convening a community task force to oversee the process. The second phase, which constituted the *assessment*, incorporated steps 2 through 5: identifying sources of information and designing research instruments (step 2), collecting data (step 3), compiling and interpreting the data (step 4), preparing and presenting the study report (step 5), and developing goals and objectives (step 6). The third phase was labeled *implementation* and contained the remaining four steps: selecting problems to work on (step 7), devising plans to decrease the severity of problems selected (step 8), implementing the plans (step 9), and evaluating the process and collecting more information where necessary (step 10). Then I presented six case studies of assessments I have been involved with.

Here I review several other models of community health needs assessment that you may find useful. Each of these is either free or available at a reasonable cost. Rather than discuss each document in entirety, my purpose is to give the orientation of each approach and then some sense of what the model involves and how to go about using it.

SOCIAL ACCOUNTABILITY BUDGETING

This approach was developed by the Catholic Health Association in conjunction with Lewin/ICF, a division of Health and Science Research Incorporated, and was the fruit of a wide-ranging group of people. The association publishes a handbook for not-for-profit healthcare providers and a separate version designed for Catholic hospitals. The approach reflects the traditional mission-driven orientation of Catholic hospitals.[1]

The preface announces it as "a set of tools for healthcare executives, professional staffs, and governing bodies to use in planning and reporting community benefits."[2] Here community health needs assessment is a part of the process of developing a "social accountability budgeting," a system for studying, evaluating, and communicating the value of the services healthcare providers furnish the community.

In the preface, William J. Cox, vice president of the Catholic Hospital Association, outlines the orientation of this approach. He sees health needs assessments as a way of resolving a "crisis of confidence" currently facing community healthcare providers.

Mr. Cox describes the crisis this way:

> We come from a tradition of community service. To a great extent our institutions were conceived out of community need, when our founders recognized the need to care for the poor and others unable to care for themselves. As time went on, our hospitals and nursing homes continued to be centers for community service, supported by community members.
>
> In recent years, however, external events have caused us to lose the closeness we once had with our communities. The Hill-Burton program helped us finance new products, and we no longer relied on community fund-raising drives for new wings and equipment. The advent of Medicare and Medicaid helped us serve the old and very poor, so our need for community financial support again lessened. But with these valuable government programs came a certain isolation from our communities—many of us stopped telling them what we were doing.
>
> Voluntary healthcare providers contribute much to our communities. We provide free charity care and numerous other services for the poor and needy. We assist with the education of health professionals and conduct medical and healthcare research. In voluntary hospitals one frequently finds services that lose money, such as burn units, and neonatal intensive care units that are provided because the community needs these services, not because they improve the bottom line.
>
> We are rarely recognized for the community services we provide. We don't provide them in order to get credit or recognition. But because these services

lack recognition, several local governments have tried (some successfully) to get hospitals and nursing homes to pay property and other taxes, claiming that these facilities are no longer charitable, but rather are healthcare businesses. Some state and local governments, seeking new revenues, are eliminating the "charitable exemption" of not-for-profit organizations, museums, and schools, as well as healthcare organizations, and are asking them to pay taxes. Some members of Congress are now questioning the business aspects of not-for-profit groups and have tried to limit the benefits of tax exemption unless hospitals are able to prove a specific charitable contribution.

Compounding this crisis of confidence is the fact that it is becoming increasingly difficult for a voluntary healthcare facility to provide community services at no charge or at a loss. Medicare margins plummeted to the point where, fiscal year 1991, we expect the majority of U.S. hospitals to lose money on most hospitals' single largest source of revenue. In most states, Medicaid payments are far below actual costs. Private insurers and businesses are demanding discounts. Further, the public is insisting that we reduce costs at the same time that we are trying to absorb the cost of caring for the growing number of persons who have no healthcare insurance at all.[3]

Mr. Cox's approach accurately stresses the pickle that he says hospitals have gotten themselves into, due to the forces of history that have walled hospitals off from the communities, and he offers social accountability budgeting as a way out. This kind of whiny, victim-thinking sort of approach becomes tiresome after a while; but, fortunately, Mr. Cox quits while he is ahead and drops the ball into the lap of Bruce Vladek, president of the United Hospital Fund of New York.

Mr. Vladek extends this analysis in the book's foreword, which is next. Sounding concepts as if they were three horses of the Apocalypse, Mr. Vladek weights community health assessment heavily with three concepts: accountability, relationship to the public, and organizational effectiveness.

Accountability

"By law and custom," Mr. Vladek begins, "publicly held corporations in the United States are accountable both to their shareholders and to a surrounding body of law designed to enforce both shareholder governance and socially acceptable behavior." Further, continues Mr. Vladek, "public agencies and institutions are . . . accountable to the public through both electoral and constitutional mechanisms." And then, the hitch: "The enforcement of accountability on private, not-for-profit institutions . . . is both more subtle and more complex." Society demands a form of accountability from hospitals as well, he continues: "certain privileges, such as a tax exemption, and enormous discretion on the understanding . . . that doing so will promote the community's ends as well as the organization's, that decisions made by the governing body will be taken with a view to the needs of the community and not just of the institution, and that such decisions will not be self-serving either in the narrow sense of self-inurement or the broader sense of institutional self-aggrandizement."

But how does the community hospital know that it has, in fact, been a good guy all along? And how does it ward off these unwarranted seizures of its assets? Here, Mr. Vladeck notes:

> Formal mechanisms for assuring institutional compliance with these expectations are limited and incomplete. An institution thus has no way of knowing, on a continuing basis, whether or not it is living up to society's expectations, or its own, unless it undertakes a process of self-examination. Doing so . . . provides a defense against unpredictable, spasmodic, and potentially quite damaging community overreaction to a perception that the institution is failing to live up to its end of the bargain."[4]

So, social accountability budgeting will help a hospital discover the extent to which it is accountable to the community. And this gives a healthcare provider a way of righting the ship that is listing too badly.

Relationship to the Public

But how do we tell the community we have been good guys, even if we know we have been? Mr. Vladek argues persuasively that such critical self-examination is "essential to building and maintaining the right kind of relationship between an institution and its community." Despite a decade of marketing, Mr. Vladek believes hospitals have not learned one important point:

> Over time, the central determinant of whether or not a hospital survives is the perception of the community(ies) it serves that it is providing an essential public service in a responsible, humane, and high quality way. For such a perception to exist in the community, the institution must carefully and consistently communicate its message over a considerable period of time. More importantly, the message it communicates must be "true."

Mr. Vladek concludes that the social accountability budget can provide a basis for communicating to the public "around which an institution can build a relationship that will stand it in good stead for years to come."

The author has made a good point; but, despite the soundness of this view, Mr. Vladek's argument reveals a basic flaw in the process—that is, the possibility that the whole process will, if placed in the wrong hands, become trivialized down to what amounts essentially to no more than another coy public relations gimmick.[5]

Organizational Effectiveness

Here is the hard part, according to Mr. Vladek:

> Unity of purpose is especially important for not-for-profit hospitals, given the broad range of professional disciplines and occupational groups they engage, the critical role of independent attending physicians, the absence of an economic "bottom line," and the very fuzziness and difficulty of defining much of what they "produce." Hospitals must thus require mechanisms for articulating and communicating a common sense of purpose around some higher end or objective; those same mechanisms provide the basis for communication both internally and externally only suggests the extent to which the purposes of well-managed hospitals and the aspirations of the public coincide."[6]

Thus, the argument made in support of this approach is that hospitals have gotten themselves into hot water, not altogether of their own making, and have become alienated from the constituents. The social accountability budgeting will enable them to understand the extent to which they have lived up to their expectations of society, will give healthcare providers a way of developing a close relationship with the communities they serve, and will promise a way of developing a strong internal culture. Further, it will enable a healthcare provider to fend off attacks on its tax-exempt status.

Social Accountability Budgeting in Action

The system itself incorporate six action areas: (1) conducting an inventory of services and activities, (2) reviewing policies and procedures, (3) taking a leadership role in needs assessments, (4) planning and budgeting for services, (5) measuring and monitoring services, and (6) reporting community benefits.

Each action area is brought to life through a series of sensible and easy-to-follow guidelines, 52 in all, listed in the table of contents. Each guideline is attractively presented and easily accessible to the reader. The handbook is liberally and effectively punctuated with neat worksheets, informational side-bars, quotes from this person and that person, and handouts useful for the reader who either wants to work through the process individually or wishes to guide his or her organization through the process.

Let's see how one of these action areas works. Take, for example, action area 10: "tak[ing] a leadership role in needs assessment."

The first guideline tells the user to "decide on the scope of the needs assessment," depending on the amount of information available in the community and whether one wishes to focus on a single aspect of care, and on the resources for conducting the assessment. Accordingly, the workbook offers a shortened or "baseline" approach and a longer "full-scale" approach. Under the baseline version, the staff in the hospital is to meet with experts in the community to review existing information, identify unmet needs, and establish a plan of action. The full-scale assessment supplements existing data with new data obtained through surveys and community forums, and it may broaden the scope of the inquiry to include all health-related needs. The first guideline comes complete with a self-appraisal worksheet.

The second guideline tells the user to form an assessment work group, a kind of ongoing brainstorming group, consisting of directors of social service and marketing, representatives of other healthcare providers or social service agencies, members of at-risk groups, and other appropriate individuals. The work group "should meet to examine existing information about health needs in the community."

The third guideline asks the work group to define the boundaries of "community." The handbook suggests that the community be defined as the area from which most of the patients come, or the area where the provider prefers that patients come from. Then the fourth guideline: "Describe the community," in terms of specific factors, such as poverty, age, minority status, non-English speaking populations, morbidity or mortality rates.

The final three guidelines lead the reader through analyzing information, collecting additional information, and collecting information from populations at risk. The discussion under this action area concludes with a model diagram of an assessment process developed by the Daughters of Charity.[7]

There are a few things I would quibble with. One of them is the consistent equating of questionnaires and surveys: "Surveys are more formal, complete questionnaires administered to members of the population at risk."[8] Not so: a questionnaire is a research tool, and a survey is a process of administering questionnaires and analyzing data so collected. And the too brief discussion of research methods is such that I wonder if many people without a research background will find it very helpful. But the handbook is comprehensive and will give you everything you wish to know. The discussion moves right along, but the time spent with it will pay off. The address given to acquire a copy is: Catholic Health Association of the United States, 4455 Woodson Road, St. Louis, Missouri 63134-3797. No phone number is provided.

HEALTHY COMMUNITIES APPROACH

Another model for community health needs assessment was developed by the National Civic League, of Denver, Colorado. Its approach is outlined in detail in a document entitled *The Healthy Communities Handbook*, published in 1993. In contrast to the Catholic Health Association's hospital-oriented approach, the National Civic League places community health in the context of healthy communities. "The solutions to many of the leading causes of sickness and premature death do not rest with our hospitals or medical service delivery systems as currently configured," writes Mr. Tyler Norris on behalf of the National Civic League. Rather,

> many of the solutions rest with our behavioral choices and those practices we encourage (or condone) as family members, neighbors, and fellow citizens. Leading health problems, such as heart disease, stroke, lung cancer, and injury from accidents, are to a great extent influenced by such choices as high fat diets and poor nutrition, lack of regular exercise, tobacco smoking, abuse of alcohol and other drugs, the failure to wear safety belts. Generally speaking, chronic and acute health conditions do not arise from lack of medical technology or access to medical professionals.

Rather, they stem from "various combinations of dysfunctional social and economic environments and a lack of access to care or appropriate intervention."[9]

Clearly, this approach is not designed to help hospitals conduct self-evaluation or to communicate better with their communities. Instead, it is designed to help people in communities work together to improve the health of their communities. It argues for "collaborative problem solving" to stimulate the efforts to improve the health status of communities. It seeks to create healthy communities by encouraging communities to redefine health and to use knowledge about the social and environmental determinants of health to find new ways to make community and family life patterns more conducive to good health.[10]

Norris argues further that people in our communities have abdicated their responsibility over their own health; "the Healthy Communities Initiative challenges individuals and communities to reclaim responsibility for their health, and to recognize that they are both the source and the beneficiary of the actions that they undertake." He concludes that "promoting the lifestyles, community standards, and policy priorities that lead to good health requires working together with the private and nonprofit sectors and with the diversity of America's population." And he adds, "those communities that recognize this need—and act collaboratively to forge a shared vision of good health—will reap the greatest benefits."[11] The authors of the handbook have intended the handbook as a "tool to help America's communities become healthier."[12]

After these introductory legions of discussions have passed by the reader, 10 chapters follow: (1) What Are Healthy Communities; (2) Assessing Community Health and the Quality of Life; (3) A Process for Creating Healthier Communities; (4) Setting the Stage—How to Begin the Healthy Communities Process; (5) (Re)Defining Health in the Community & Environmental Scan; (6) Evaluating Current Realities and Trends; (7) Developing a Healthy Community Vision & Selecting and Evaluating Key Performance Areas; (8) Creating the Action Plan & Implementation Strategy; (9) Project Implementation and (10) The Community Outreach Process. A number of appendixes bring up the rear, one entitled "Tools and Models," one giving more information about the National Civic League, a third listing public health resources, a fourth describing health indicators, and a bibliography.

The first chapter discusses concepts of a healthy community and collaborative problem solving, defines the notion of "community," specifies the characteristics of a healthy community, and gives some examples of programs that promote healthy communities. Collaborative problem solving is described in this chapter pretty much as it was in the foreword, as a "problem-solving process that allows a broad spectrum of community stakeholders to create a vision of health and implement a plan to turn its vision into reality,"[13] as a process that will result in specific positive outcomes, conveniently itemized in a "bullet" list.

The discussion of community here is not particularly insightful. We learn only that (1) the concept of community is difficult to define, that (2) many people define it differently in different places, and that (3) a community must encompass a defined geographic area. The chapter continues by listing 6 elements of healthy cities, 11 model characteristics of a healthy city, and 14 elements of a healthy community, none of which any reasonable person would quarrel with.[14]

Finally, the chapter lists a series of state, national, and international healthy city programs from which users can learn. Local programs listed include: KidsPlace, Seattle, Washington; Winchester–Frederick County, Virginia; UrbanCare, South Bend, Indiana; Community Partners, Coalition Building for Local Service Delivery Systems, Boston, Massachusetts; Palm Desert, California; Monterey Park, California. State, national, and international programs listed include: The United States Healthy Communities Initiative; Healthy People 2000; Building Healthier Communities, the United Way; Colorado Healthy Communities Initiative; California Healthy Cities Project; Promoting Healthy Traditions; Wellness Councils of America (WELCOA); and WHO–International Healthy Cities. Each program is briefly described and a contact person is listed.[15]

The second chapter, "Assessing Community Health and Quality of Life," explores the value of developing a community profile and monitoring the health and quality of life indicators. The handbook describes a profile as "a set of key community health indicators which assist in setting priorities and documenting the success or relative success of a given project."[16] Examples of indicators given are "infant mortality rate; incidence of death from coronary heart disease; rate of lung cancer death; death rates for alcohol-related motor vehicle accidents; rates of teen pregnancy; and rates of low birthweight babies."[17] The author gives a number of guidelines for evaluating the desirability of specific indicators—validity, timeliness, stability, reliability, understandability, responsiveness, policy relevance and representativeness—and gives a range of various kinds of indicators and sources where they may be found.[18]

The third chapter lays out the heart of the National Civic League's process of creating healthier communities. After commenting on the importance of collaboration and listing several keys to success, the process is outlined in some detail.

The process flows through two phases: planning and implementation. Planning incorporates seven steps: beginning the process by bringing together a team of initiators, or project "champions"; launching the effort by coming to consensus on the definition of health; conducting an "environmental scan," which assists the community in defining major issues;

evaluating current trends in community health and the quality of life and the capacity of the community to solve its problems; developing a "healthy community vision"; evaluating "key performance areas," or themes on which the group can hang the process; and creating an action plan and implementation strategy.

The second phase initiates the implementation of the process in three steps: shifting from planning to implementation by selecting a lead implementation team of people to move the process along, selecting a group that will carry on, and monitoring any changes in the community that may have occurred since the project was begun.[19]

The remaining chapters focus on selected aspects of the process laid out in the third chapter. I found the section on developing a healthy community vision particularly interesting. The process defines a vision as "an expression of possibility—an ideal future state that the community might hope to attain."[20] The handbook lays out some basic pointers in developing a vision; that is, it should be (1) stated in positive terms, (2) expressed in easily understood language, (3) set within a reasonable time period, (4) focused on people and the quality of life, (5) and so forth. The handbook continues to lay out a process model for the "visioning process": warming up the group in a large group setting, breaking down into smaller groups that report back, and so forth. The handbook goes into great depth, which I will not attempt to summarize. But by now I am sure you get the picture.

The handbook is very clear, well written, informative, accessible, and—and this is the best part—entertaining. However, knowing the community consensus process as I do, I would be loathe to undertake the process. Democracy is a wonderful yet inefficient process, and getting powerful groups to work together in a sustained effort over a period of a decade seems chimerical to me. My experience has told me that consensus building will work only when either engineered from the top or if a small band of fiercely dedicated fanatical community workers pushed ahead, willing to ignore the opposition of significant portions of the community that opposed them.

I also found myself quibbling with the author's understanding of research methods. For example, in Chapter 10, "The Community Outreach Process," the author discusses focus groups: "Focus groups are a form of survey." They aren't a survey. Further, he says "focus groups are time-consuming and usually take up to a minimum of one month to assemble and conduct." Wrong again. Focus groups can be assembled and conducted in as quickly as two weeks, if done right. Third, he says "the focus group leader must make sure the groups are representative of the demographics within the community to ensure a valid sampling of perspectives." Well, as I note in my chapter on research methods, focus groups are used in qualitative research, an area of research to which notions of sampling and validity are inapplicable.[21] To the author's credit, he notes that this discussion is very brief and that users should consult or perhaps hire a professional researcher. One of my underlying themes is that needs assessments are essentially research processes, and that those who do them must have either research skills themselves or access to others with sound research skills.

Despite my qualms, this process is well laid out, has a lot to recommend it, has a lot of success stories to which it can point, and can be very helpful to people interested in mobilizing community resources. The handbook is available through the National Civics League, 1445 Market Street, Suite 300, Denver, Colorado 80302-1728. The league's phone number is (303) 571-4343.

APEX/PH

A third model for assessing the health of a community is *APEX* (Assessment Protocol for Excellence in Public Health), published in 1991. The manual tells us that the process began in July 1987 as a cooperative project of the American Public Health Association, the Centers for Disease Control and Prevention, and several other public health agencies. In developing the process, APHA and others subjected the workbook to extensive field tests at 13 demonstration sites, "selected to include large, medium, and small health departments."[22]

The process is outlined in a thick workbook, intended for use by local health department officials. The process was designed to help public health officials enhance "their organizational capacity and strengthen their leadership role in their communities." The workbook covers two main areas: "(1) assessing and improving the organizational capacity of the department and (2) working with the local community to assess and improve the health status of citizens." The details of the two areas are filled in three parts: "organizational capacity assessment," "community process," and "completing the cycle."

The first section of the manual, which discusses organizational capacity, shows officials how to assess the capabilities of their organization, develop an organizational work plan, and set priorities to "correct perceived weaknesses." I assume that some effort will be made to make sure perceived weaknesses are real weaknesses.

The second section, which discusses the community process, "strengthens the partnership between a local health department and its community in addressing the community's major public health problems and building a healthier community," exhorting the user to form a community advisory committee and to set health status goals and programmatic objectives in order to "mobilize community resources in pursuit of locally relevant public health objectives."

The third section, "Completing the Cycle," focuses on activities necessary to carry out activities in the first two sections. It covers policy development, assurance, monitoring, and evaluation.[23]

Here we have a third view of who should take the lead in addressing community health status. According to the Catholic Health Association model, the local hospital should do it. According to the National Civic League model, the citizenry should do it. Here we have folks saying the public health department should do it:

> If we, as a society, are to improve the conditions that affect the health of all of us, we must begin in local communities, dealing with local conditions. Local health departments have a responsibility to take a key role in this effort. They should lead their communities in an examination of local health problems and in the development of plans to overcome those problems. This workbook provides a process by which a local health department can assume this leadership role and work with its community toward a common goal of improved health for its citizens.[24]

In the following text, the key role of public health is further elaborated as follows. Administering a public health department is a really, really big job. It is hard to step back and take a look at the organization to evaluate it and make it more responsive to the community. But, because "government has a basic duty to assure the public's health," officials must take time for it. Because public health problems "require hard choices," public health departments must bite the bullet. With accountability comes leadership, and health departments must set and meet standards of competence and practice that are seen as relevant to the community. Because public health problems are deep-seated and multidimensional and because improvements in public health require coordinated responses and active community ownership and commitment, public health departments must find ways to work in partnership with their communities, to provide their communities with scientific health information, and to seek creative solutions from a wide range of community resources.[25]

The first part of the process covers conducting an organizational capacity assessment. A nicely laid out flow chart lists the following steps: (1) preparing for organizational capacity assessment, (2) scoring indicators for importance and current status, (3) identifying strengths and weaknesses, (4) analyzing and reporting strengths, (5) analyzing weaknesses, (6) ranking problems in order of priority, (7) developing and implementing action plans, and (8) institutionalizing the assessment process.[26] The workbook clearly discusses each step; it is readable and useful and provides some very handy worksheets.

Now I visualize that you will ask me why this should be important for you, because it is about local health department officials. Strictly speaking, this is true. However, the process is a sound one for analyzing any organization, and, in most cases, the reader can freely substitute the word *hospital* for that of *public health department* without a stir. In other words, you can use this process to analyze your own organization's capacities for conducting community health assessment. In fact, almost any organization could use it to analyze organizational capacity for almost any area of endeavor.

The second part of the manual focuses on community involvement and, perhaps, deserves a little more attention. The *APEX*/PH community process is also laid out in a concise flow chart: (1) preparing for the community process, (2) collecting and analyzing health data, (3) forming a community health committee, (4) identifying community health problems, (5) prioritizing community health problems, (6) analyzing community health problems, and (7) developing a community health plan.[27]

To supplement the flow charts and worksheets, in the appendixes one finds useful items: descriptions of the methodologies used at test sites; procedures to use by a policy board in scoring indicators; model job descriptions for community health committee members; model bylaws for a community health committee; a method for setting priorities among health problems; a self-assessment form for use by a community health committee; a resource bibliography; references; and a glossary.[28]

Note clearly that, because this model is developed from a public sector orientation, its approach to community involvement is essentially "top down." It sees government as the primary caretaker of the public good. Its methodology for community health planning is limited largely to recruiting community people by the public health agency. Data to be collected are secondary only, available from published sources. I will say more about secondary and primary research in Chapter Eight.

Secondary data should be examined before collecting any primary data is contemplated. If secondary data are valid, timely, and specific to your community, by all means use them. It is usually less expensive, quicker, and easier to rely on the published sources, such as local or state health departments, the CDC, and federal agencies. Often, however, published sources are either limited or entirely inadequate, because they are outdated or unreliable or not relevant to the community to be assessed. In some cases, those who need the data may not be able to find the information they need, or they may need information faster than it can be obtained from published sources. If this is the case, you will need to collect some primary data using a standard social science research method, usually some kind of focus group study or survey. This workbook will be of no use to you in this regard.

Nevertheless, this process is a sound one and does well at what it is intended to do. It can be obtained from the National Association of County Health Officials, 440 First Street, N.W., Washington, D.C. 20001.

PATCH

A fourth process reviewed here is PATCH, which stands for Planned Approach to Community Health, developed during the 1980s by the Centers for Disease Control and Prevention in partnership with state and local health departments and community groups. Here is how the CDC describes PATCH:

> The Planned Approach to Community Health (PATCH) is a methodology that many communities use to plan, conduct, and evaluate health promotion and disease prevention programs. The process helps a community establish a health promotion team, collect and use local data, set health priorities, design interventions, and evaluate their effect. Adaptable to a variety of situations, the PATCH planning process can be used when a community wants to identify and address priority health problems or when the health priority or special population to be addressed has already been selected. It can also be adapted and used by existing organizational and planning structures in the community.

The initial goal of PATCH was to improve communities' capacity to plan, implement, and evaluate comprehensive community-based health promotion activities targeted toward priority health problems.[29]

Five elements define the PATCH process. First, active participation by a wide range of community members is fundamental to the process. These members plan, set priorities, and make all programmatic decisions. Second, data drive the development of programs. Analysis of local and other data sources "are analyzed to guide the selection of health priorities, as well as program development and evaluation." Third, once community members become involved and data are analyzed, and once community policies, services, and resources are reviewed, "an overall community health promotion strategy is designed." Interventions that encourage changing destructive behaviors and maintaining constructive behaviors are conducted in schools, healthcare facilities, community centers and churches, the workplace, and other appropriate community sites. Fourth, we have feedback and improvement: timely feedback and evaluation help people monitor their progress and make improvements in their programs.

The fifth concept assumes that through this process the capacity of the community for health promotion is increased. This effect is explained as follows:

> PATCH is an ongoing process that can be used to address a variety of health priorities. PATCH aims to cultivate community health planning and health promotion skills and resources with a community so that the mechanisms for addressing future activities are put in place. It also encourages the community to establish partnerships with organizations and groups beyond the community."[30]

The PATCH process is organized in five stages. The first is "mobilizing the community . . . an ongoing process that starts in phase I as a community organizes to begin PATCH and continues throughout the PATCH process." During this first phase, "the community is defined, participants are recruited from the community, and a demographic profile of the community is completed. . . . The community group and steering committee are then organized and working groups are created." The second phase begins "when community members form working groups to obtain and analyze data on mortality, morbidity, community opinion, and behaviors." Members analyze data, determine the leading health problems, and devise ways of sharing the results of the data analysis with the community. During the third phase, "choosing health priorities," the "additional data collected are presented to the community group. The group analyzes the behavioral, social, economic, political, and environmental factors that affect behaviors that put people at risk for disease, disability, and injury." To my mind, this one isn't very clearly distinguished from the second phase, and I am not sure that community participants have the skills to do these things; but I think the picture is clear enough to give you the flavor of the thing. The fourth phase is "developing a comprehensive intervention strategy." According to the model, "The community group chooses, designs, and conducts interventions . . . and devises a comprehensive health promotion strategy, sets intervention objectives, and develops an intervention plan." The whole idea behind this part is that "throughout, members of the target groups are involved in the process of planning interventions." Phase V is an evaluation phase, ongoing, designed to monitor and assess progress during the five phases of PATCH and to evaluate the interventions.

The CDC has published a guide to about 74 PATCH projects around the country, and it includes a page-long description of each project, together with names and addresses of the coordinators for each project. The information available to me looks rather incomplete. When I called the PATCH office, I was told that the document was in the process of being printed. I asked them to send me the most current information, and from them I received a program summary, two chapters labeled "draft" from their concept guide, a document entitled PATCH Meeting Guide, which includes a lot of training material for PATCH coordinators, a stapled volume of checklists, a sample interview schedule for a community survey, and some worksheets.

From the materials on my desk, it is hard to see how a community could pull this off unless it has a dedicated cadre of volunteer and community coordinators to move the process along. Nevertheless, the program is widely used, so they must be doing something right. Also, I think that the survey materials enclosed are insufficient, and if I were someone in the community facing this process, I would feel overwhelmingly daunted. But, for more information on PATCH, you can write to the Division of Chronic Disease Control and Community Intervention, National Center for Chronic Disease Control and Prevention, Mailstop K-46, 4770 Buford Highway, N.E., Atlanta, Georgia 30341. Call (404) 488-5426, or fax them at (404) 488-5964.

MODEL STANDARDS APPROACH

This approach encourages local leaders to "engage a whole host of players in setting the health priorities for their locales" to implement programs to achieve health objectives. The model standards approach builds on this perspective, and the handbook, at about 500 pages, is the thickest of all the books reviewed here.[31]

The authors begin: "During the 1980s, national leaders recognized that improvements in health status require efforts targeted to people in communities where they live." The authors then list three elements involved in translating national objectives into "achievable community health targets": (1) an "understandable set of health status and local process objectives that can be readily measured"; (2) readily available "strategies to achieve these objectives involving public, private, and voluntary sectors of the community"; and (3) a "coordinating process to help ensure that the community can work together."[32]

The *APEX*/PH approach viewed the public sector as the key actor in preserving the health status of the community, and the model standards approach agrees. It reaffirms that public health agencies are the "final delivery point for all public health efforts," and they are responsible for leadership that fosters local responsibility and "equitably distributing public resources and private activities."[33]

The chapter entitled "How to Use Model Standards" outlines the approach. It encourages readers to use the objectives spelled out in its companion handbook, *Healthy People 2000*, as a basis for community health planning. The *Healthy People 2000* objectives have been "adapted verbatim" for this approach.

The chapter then lists eight model standards principles: (1) emphasis on health outcomes—that is, using as "guiding stars" a set of measurable and realistic targets; (2) flexibility for local communities to adapt goals to reflect local conditions; (3) focus on the entire community, to facilitate community groups and agencies to work together; (4) government as the "residual guarantor," so "every locale and population served [will be] served by a unit of government that takes a leadership role in assuring the public's health"; (5) importance of negotiation in promoting agreement among agencies and individuals who have an interest in improving public health; (6) standards to ensure uniform objectives "to assure equity and social justice" and guidelines to emphasize "local discretion for decision-making"; (7) accessibility of services to help communities tailor special targets to those most in need; and (8) emphasis on programs to avoid over-reliance on professional practice standards.[34] Anyone approaching community health assessment from either a community or hospital focus will pause longer over the concept of government as the guarantor of the public's health.

After discussing a few examples of local "success stories," the chapter goes on to list "activities for implementation," all summarized in a side-bar: (1) assessment of the role of one's health agency; (2) assessment of the lead health agency's organizational capacity; (3) devel-opment of an agency plan, to build the necessary organizational capacity; (4) assessing the community's organizational and power structures; (5) organizing the community, to build a stronger constituency for public health and estab-lish a partnership for public health; (6) assessing the health needs and available community resources; (7) determining local priorities; (8) selecting outcome and process objectives; (9) developing communitywide intervention strategies; (10) development and implementation of a plan of action; (11) monitoring and evaluating the effort on a continuing basis.[35]

Anyone who has read the description of or who has used the *APEX*/PH manual will understand that this handbook is very similar. In fact, *Healthy Communities 2000* refers to *APEX*/PH as offering a structured way of car-rying out the activities listed in the book. In fact, the chapter continues to describe each step in greater detail, descriptions which I won't go into here. The chapter ends with a summary and a brief description of how to develop community-based targets.[36]

The handbook then lists goals and objectives in 26 separate areas, rang-ing from physical activity and fitness to diabetes and chronic disabling conditions. In each topic area, the handbook provides a focused health sta-tus objective, such as "weapon-related violent deaths," and an indicator for planners to use in determining whether each has met the objective. Along with each objective are some baseline data to assist in determining the date at which the objective is to be reached. The objectives are quite wide rang-ing. For example, under the topic "violent and abusing behavior" are listed 37 separate objectives. Anyone picking up the handbook may find this rather daunting. Nevertheless, the handbook is quite complete and useful.

STATE HOSPITAL ASSOCIATION MODELS

Finally, I wish to review several guidebooks developed by state hospital associations kind enough to share them with me. I tried to look at some from others such as VHA and Sun Health, but they would not return my telephone calls. Missouri has developed a manual but did not make it available to me. So you will have to contact those organizations yourself if you wish to consider them.

Wisconsin

The Wisconsin Hospital Association's *Community Collaboration for Health; a Guide to Building Healthier Communities* has just become available. It was primarily the work of Mr. Paul Zak, a graduate student in healthcare policy and administration at the University of Wisconsin–Madison. It is essentially a distillation of other manuals put together in a very useful, attractive, and entertaining way. The manual starts out this way:

> The developments and changes in the healthcare sector in recent years have combined to generate a paradigm shift in the way hospitals and other healthcare providers think about, manage, and deliver healthcare. Hospitals have traditionally operated in a model of healthcare that focuses on acute care services and treating illnesses. Increasingly, however, hospitals and health systems are being challenged to operate on a public health model of promoting wellness and explicitly demonstrating accountability for maximizing community health and minimizing costs. In addition to their traditional acute care and clinical treatment roles, there are increasing calls for hospitals to include services oriented toward promotion of healthy lifestyles wellness, and disease prevention. Indeed, the future of healthcare, and the success (even survival) of healthcare providers, will be driven by efforts to design and implement initiatives aimed at assessing and improving the health of a broad population.
>
> This document emphasizes the importance of adopting an expanded, comprehensive definition of health which moves beyond medical/clinical factors to address the psycho-social and environmental determinants of a person's well-being. Operating from this definition, the document explains how hospitals can and should participate in and/or facilitate a communitywide collaboration that will coordinate human, physical, and financial resources to assess community health needs, set goals and priorities, develop efficient and effective health improvement strategies, and implement intervention programs to address needs and improve community health status in measurable ways.[37]

The document gives three main "foci" in community health assessment. First, it takes a "strategic focus," to address the strategic reasons why hospitals need to participate in community health assessment initiatives, specifically as a planning tool to "help hospitals capitalize on the opportunities to meet specific challenges." As you can see, this process is a hospital-focused process. Second, it incorporates a "conceptual" focus, to stress the need for a broader definition of health and the need for collaboration among community groups. It sees this collaborative process as an extension of continuous quality improvement methods. Third, it brings to the table a "process and implementation focus, incorporating a six-step model adapted from a variety of existing health assessment tools and publications."[38]

The six phases of the Wisconsin model are these. First, ensuring a hospital's commitment and capacity, in which "the appropriate commitment, capacity, motivation, resources, and vision . . . are mobilized and consolidated and a structure is set in place within the hospital to monitor its involvement in the collaborative health improvement process." The second phase has as its goal to "initiate and structure a communitywide partnership that works together in a systematic and coordinated fashion to define the community and profile its health status." Third, a partnership profiles the community by "obtaining, organizing, and analyzing data on a variety of key health status indicators, including quantitative measures . . . and qualitative measures," and renders those data understandable in the form of tables, charts, and graphs, "matching the summarized data to preselected criteria." The fourth phase considers those issues identified during the last phase and addresses those it selects with intervention programs or projects. During phase five, intervention programs or projects across a number of priority areas are designed and implemented. Finally, phase six is an evaluation, in which both the product and the process are critiqued. In summary, the Wisconsin Hospital Association recommends that hospitals use its guide to help them accomplish the following: redefine health more broadly, reexamine their mission or vision statements, initiate collaborative health planning efforts, develop community health plans, and apply continuous quality improvement principles and processes to the healthier community effort.

The guide is organized in 10 parts. The first outlines clearly and persuasively why hospitals should do community health assessment, and the second part defines what community health assessment is, though not quite as persuasively. The next six sections lay out in greater detail each of the six steps outlined above. The final section consists of eight appendixes, consisting of useful worksheets, data sources, community profiles, case studies, and a glossary of terms.

The manual achieves a nice balance between coverage and depth. It never stays too long in one place, but never leaves the reader behind. It is very well written and attractively presented and gives lots of references to other guidebooks and sources. Nevertheless, to implement this process requires the user to invest a considerable amount of sweat equity. To obtain a copy, contact Ms. Marsha Borling, RN, Wisconsin Hospital Association,

5721 Odana Road, Madison, Wisconsin 53719-1289. Call (608) 274-1820; fax (608) 274-8554.

Pennsylvania

The Hospital Association of Pennsylvania has been a leader in promoting community health needs assessments. Its guide was kindly made available to me by the association so I could review it for this book. It is the best known and probably the skimpiest—and probably the least desirable— from my perspective, anyway. Much, I think, is misleading, and I disagree with much of it. But, let's see what we can make of it.

The guidebook began as an effort to provide attendees at a training seminar with information about areas where their hospitals are located. In its final form, it evolved into a major project for the Committee on Health Care Data and the Policy Research Department of the Hospital Association of Pennsylvania.[39]

For a theme it quotes a verse inscribed on a stone monument built in memory of Johnny Appleseed, who "planted seeds that others might enjoy fruit." The association consciously selected the apple image as a symbol of health and well-being, and it developed the guidebook around the concept to emphasize the transition from a seed to the development of a mature tree. Leaving aside the appropriateness of a metaphor about apple tree planting and the question of whether there ever was a Johnny Appleseed, the HAP manual states its orientation in this way:

> As the nation prepares for healthcare reform, communities are becoming the center of attention and focal point to effect change. . . . This effort is complemented by increasing calls to seriously recognize and address the overall health needs of our population.
>
> In sum, the future will be driven by programs emphasizing preventive services and implementing initiatives aimed at assessing and improving our health status. To that end, the *Healthy People 2000* consortium, facilitated by the Institute of Medicine of the National Academy of Sciences as assisted by the U.S. Public Health Services, using a series of work groups of national expertise, developed three aggressive national goals: increase the span of healthy lives for Americans, reduce health disparities among Americans, and achieve access to preventative services for all Americans.
>
> In Pennsylvania, the Hospital Association of Pennsylvania (HAP), working with a panel of healthcare leaders, embarked on an ambitious effort to serve as a catalyst for change through a vision of the future of healthcare in this state.

HAP's vision focuses on opportunities to create partnerships for action based on the resources, the desires and the motivation of communities to identify their own healthcare priorities. The underlying values that support this vision are: we believe that all Pennsylvanians must have access to appropriate and necessary care; we believe that healthcare in Pennsylvania must be affordable; we believe that improvements in health status of Pennsylvanians must be the primary measure of our success; we believe that the healthcare system must continue to accommodate the cultural diversity of our society; we recognize our fundamental responsibility for working in partnership with other members of the nation's human service system to enhance the quality of life; we recognize our responsibility to sustain an ongoing commitment to continuous improvement.[40]

The association designed the guide to serve as both a companion document for the county health profile as well as a tool to help communities do the following: "learn and understand . . . what makes communities unique"; recognize that "information characterizing the health behavior of a community, a comprehensive inventory of human services agencies, and an appreciation for the economic impact of healthcare in a community provide an invaluable insight into the pervasive nature of healthcare"; work together, "drawing on the perceptions, expertise, and support of local resources, to establish a list of needs, priorities, and targets for attention"; "rally" the community to develop aggressive action plans and interventions; and "measure and assess the impact that community action has on the health status of the population and to continually strive to improve its effectiveness."

The authors of the guide stress that it is not a detailed "cookbook." Rather, it is "set up to give the reader a sense of how information collected from a variety of sources and methods can be used effectively to stimulate a community to take a positive step toward community-defined goals and objectives. In fact, as you read through this process, each section contains less detail, relying instead on community input and action."[41]

The HAP model incorporates five phases. The first phase consists of constructing a county profile, which presents summary information designed to illustrate the characteristics of the community. According to the guide, "the seed of the healthcare profiles, when germinated through introduction to the community, should stimulate local leaders to collect other information to complete a Community Health Assessment."[42] The second phase tries to show how a community currently perceives itself in terms of human behaviors, inventories of health and human resources, and the impact that all of these elements have on the community. The third phase shows how the community can begin to organize itself through a series of focus groups, how the groups can be conducted, and how the results can be summarized. I will have more to say about this part later. The fourth phase describes and offers suggestions regarding how community leaders can come together to formulate a definitive action plan. "This phase represents an apple tree fully maturing and flowering, waiting for the course of time to bear fruit." Finally, phase five incorporates assessing, analyzing, identifying, and prioritizing.[43]

The first section covers county health profiles in some detail and focuses on questions to ask concerning demographic characteristics of the community, healthcare resources, and health status indicators. It has a brief but very clear discussion of health status indicators, and I learned from it that Pennsylvania seems to have county-specific indicators. These data are very useful in evaluating the health status of an area.

The second section recommends conducting a "personal behavior survey," based on the CDC Behavior Risk Factor Survey conducted through the state department of health. We use this survey routinely and find it a valid research tool, because it produces data that can be compared with statewide data as well as against *Healthy People 2000* goals. The guide recommends conducting a mailed survey, 5,000 questionnaires strong, complemented by a telephone survey. The reasons for selecting this methodology are not clearly spelled out, and the guide indicates that the mailed questionnaire will have a response rate of 15 percent, which is too low to be valid. In addition, it recommends 300 telephone surveys to test the sampling distribution of the mailed questionnaire. In my view, a random household telephone survey is sufficient, but it may require more than 300 completed interviews. If you are going to conduct a mailed survey, sound practice is to test the results. However, whether a sample size of 300 is recommended depends on the situation.

The discussion argues for computer analysis of research results via statistical software, use of appropriate statistical tests, and presentation graphics. This provides support for my argument that, to conduct research, you should use qualified research professionals, not volunteers. These tools of the trade are most commonly found in research companies and university research facilities. I will take issue with one more point. In developing the inventory of resources, the guide recommends that the steering committee develop a survey to be used. Again, my strong argument is that researchers are needed to design surveys (not steering committees).

The third phase argues for a focus group approach, to allow people to express their opinions and to speak out. As I discuss later in this book, focus groups, in my opinion, are the wrong approach. Hold a series of town meetings. Let people speak out at community forums. Conduct brainstorming sessions and have nominal groups at these meetings. Fine, but not focus groups. And even if, and that is *if*, focus group were appropriate, the instructions in the guide would not help you conduct one successfully.

The final phases cover the ground well and offer some help in thinking about the process. I will quibble, though, with the notion that a plan is definitive. No plan is definitive. It should be a living, breathing entity, not an inscription in stone. Every plan needs to be constantly reevaluated and changed as necessary.

The guide contains two appendixes. The first appendix consists of data sources, a glossary, a small area variation analysis, DRG Cross-Reference Listings, and a map of Pennsylvania. The second appendix purports to show the reader how to read tables and charts. I must confess, if I didn't know how to read them, that explanation wouldn't help much.

You can get hold of one of these guides by contacting Mr. John Hope, vice president of Communication Services, the Hospital Association of Pennsylvania, 4750 Lindle Road, P.O. Box 8600, Harrisburg, PA 17105-8600. Call (717) 561-5335.

Kansas

The last process I will review in this chapter is the CHAP process, devised jointly by three organizations: the Kansas Department of Health and Environment, the Kansas Hospital Association, and the Kansas Association of Local Health Departments. CHAP stands for Community Health Assessment Process. What I received was a bound 35-page document, subtitled "Overview," and a weighty three-ring binder, entitled "Workbook." Just picking up the workbook is a healthy behavior. The "overview" gives the highlights of the process, and the workbook gives details.

As I have said, the three organizations listed above developed CHAP working together. The authors state that, in developing the model, "proven community health assessment processes, such as PATCH (Planned Approach to Community Health) and *APEX*/PH (Advanced Protocol for Excellence in Public Health), have been reviewed, and the most appropriate resources and concepts have been modified to fit the diverse needs of

Kansas communities."[44] The authors state at the outset that the long-term goal of CHAP is to "improve and promote the health of community members by: educating community members regarding healthy behaviors; attacking the risks which contribute to the leading causes of death, disability; and improving the health services delivery system." The authors further emphasize that "CHAP is a process, not a one-time event."[45] According to the authors, this long-term goal is achieved through a process that is community controlled, comprehensive, and data-driven.

To pause for a second, it is a subtle thing but note that the stated goal is to improve the health of "community members," not of the community as a whole. This strikes me as a case of sloppy writing, because, if this process were to focus on individuals, rather than on the community at large, it would ignore environmental health altogether as irrelevant. The rest of the document does not ignore environmental issues, so here I am, wishing that the thing had been given another editing.

Involved in the process is a mix of three kinds of data: data on health status risks, on healthcare systems, and on community perception. The first kind, sloppily referred to as "health status risks," includes data on maternal and child health, morbidity, mortality, behavioral risks, demographics, socioeconomics, environmental risks, and crime. Although the examples given are related to health risk behaviors, the casualness with which the terms are used sounds as though the terms are words the author has heard about but not quite understood. Second, "Health Care System data includes [sic] information relating to services provided in the community and other healthcare system issues. Example types of Health Care System data are: health services, social services, environmental health services, health networks, transportation, financial resources, and human resources." Did you notice the incorrect agreement of "includes" with "data," and the poor usage of "Example types" above? This kind of imprecise usage and poor writing flaws this document. Well, let's go on. The third kind of data is labeled "community perceptions." Again, note the incorrect usage: "Community perceptions data can include all sources of community opinion relating to health issues." The author includes the following as "sources of community perception": a representative CHAP team, provider and consumer questionnaires, health organization satisfaction surveys, opinion surveys, town meetings, focus groups, and community workshops. Actually, these are not sources of community perceptions, they are areas through which community perceptions can be sampled with some survey approach. Most readers will know what they mean, despite the fuzzy language. Finally, the introduction points out a list of things in the workbook, which is definitely worth checking out.

After this rather inept introduction, the overview lays out a six-phase process. The first five phases are supposed to take six months, the remaining phase will be ongoing. The first phase is spent "involving and educating your community." The major tasks to be accomplished during this phase are assembling the CHAP team, involving any outside consultants or others with expertise, and informing the community. Once the CHAP team is in place, and the community is oriented, the second phase begins. This phase is called "Reviewing Community Data," in which the CHAP team reviews existing data from public sources and constructs a health profile of the community. This serves as a kind of starting point. The third phase involves "collecting community data." This "community data" includes taking stock of the resources of the community and conducting an opinion survey of the community. The authors rightly recommend that outside assistance should be sought in the survey process. Once you have finished this part, the manual says you have finished the hardest part. I think you have just finished the easiest part. The hard part is getting things accomplished once the assessment process is completed. The fourth phase is referred to as "understanding your community's data," and serves as a bridge between reviewing data and developing the community health plan, a process of pulling together all the health status, perceptual, and other data you have collected. The fifth phase, then, is devoted to developing the community plan, called the most important part of CHAP. The authors warn the reader not to take on too much, and this is very good advice. As they correctly point out, this is an ongoing process, and you can take on new objectives as time goes on. The sixth phase involves implementing the plan and evaluating CHAP. To me, this is the hardest part. All of the fanfare is over and the adrenaline rush of planning, analysis, and research is over. Now, digging the trenches begins, and those persistent volunteers must be found to accomplish the tasks planned. This, briefly discussed, is the process in general terms. The rest of the overview document gives some flow charts and describes the process in some additional detail. For the guts of the project, the reader must lift and open the workbook, which, as I noted above, is no mean feat.

The workbook is very detailed and useful. It has a wealth of information about the health status of Kansas, and lots of checklists and worksheets to help the user. There is a small amount of advice for conducting research. What they say is accurate, but not enough is really useful without seeking outside help.

In short, this is a competent process, though I wish the manual had been less conceptually fuzzy. You can get a copy by writing the the Kansas Department of Health and Environment at 900 SW Jackson, Suite 665, Topeka, Kansas 66612-1290, or call (913) 296-1200.

IN SUM

Reviewing these processes left me feeling a little like I had just sampled wallpaper. Each sheet has a slightly different pattern, but all of them cover the same area. And the selection of one over another finally comes down, in the final analysis, to a matter of taste and what you want to spend.

ENDNOTES

1. Trocchio, Julie; Timothy Eckles; and Keith Hearle et al. *Social Accountability Budget for Not-for-Profit Healthcare Organizations.* (St. Louis: Catholic Hospital Association, 1989).
2. Trocchio, *Social Accountability Budget*, p. vii.
3. Trocchio, *Social Accountability Budget*, pp. vii–viii.
4. Trocchio, *Social Accountability Budget*, pp. ix–x.
5. Trocchio, *Social Accountability Budget*, p. x.
6. Trocchio, *Social Accountability Budget*, p. x.
7. Trocchio, *Social Accountability Budget*, pp. 23–33.
8. Trocchio, *Social Accountability Budget*, p. 31.
9. Norris, Tyler. *The Healthy Communities Handbook.* Denver: National Civic League, 1993, pp. v–vi.
10. Norris, p. vi.
11. Norris, p. vii.
12. Norris, p. 3.
13. Norris, p. 6.
14. Norris, pp. 8–10.
15. Norris, pp. 11–25.
16. Norris, p. 26.

17. Norris, p. 27.

18. Norris, pp. 27–42

19. Norris, pp. 46–64.

20. Norris, p. 89.

21. Norris, pp. 104–5.

22. *APEX: Assessment Protocol for Excellence in Public Health.* Washington, D.C.: National Association of County Health Officials, 1991), pp. 6, 7.

23. *APEX,* p. iii.

24. *APEX,* p. 3.

25. *APEX,* pp. 3–4.

26. *APEX,* p. 10.

27. *APEX,* p. 78.

28. *APEX,* p. 168ff.

29. *Planned Approach to Community Health (PATCH): Program Descriptions.* Washington, D.C.: U.S. Department of Health and Human Services, 1993, p. i.

30. *PATCH,* pp. iii.

31. *Healthy Communities 2000: Model Standards. Guidelines for Community Attainment of the Year 2000 National Health Objectives.* 3d ed. Washington D.C.: American Public Health Association, 1991, pp. vii, viii.

32. *Healthy Communities 2000,* p. viii.

33. *Healthy Communities 2000,* p. ix.

34. *Healthy Communities 2000,* pp. viii, ix.

35. *Healthy Communities 2000,* p. xxii.

36. *Healthy People 2000,* pp. xxvii, xxviii.

37. Zak, Paul; Marsha Borling; and Marvin Kolb. *Community Collaboration for Health; a Guide for Building Healthier Communities.* Madison: Wisconsin Hospital Association, 1995, p. 3.

38. Zak, *Community Collaboration for Health,* pp. 3, 4.

39. *A Guide for Assessing and Improving Health Status; Community . . . Planting the Seeds for Good Health.* Hospital Association of Pennsylvania, 1993.

40. HAP, *A Guide,* pp. 3, 4

41. HAP, *A Guide,* p. 2.

42. HAP, *A Guide,* p. 4.

43. HAP, *A Guide,* p. 4.

44. *Kansas Community Health Assessment Process (CHAP); Overview.* Topeka: Kansas Department of Health and Environment, 1995, p. Intro-A-1.

45. *CHAP Overview,* p. Intro-A-2.

Chapter Nine

Research Tips

INTRODUCTION

Assessing the health needs of your community requires research. As I have noted before, several times, you should use a research team, or at least retain a research professional to assist you. No steering committees, no volunteer task forces—please. You should no more use a volunteer accountant to do an appendectomy than you should use a nonresearcher to conduct research. Enough of that. But if you aren't persuaded by this, and you wish to go ahead anyway, I have included some tips to save you from basic errors. Or, if you are already involved in a project and want to become more knowledgeable about research, this chapter will help you.

FIRST, WHAT WE ARE TALKING ABOUT

What Is Research?

Research, according to Webster, involves investigation, inquiry, scrutiny, and examination. Specifically, research is defined as the "careful, systematic, diligent inquiry or examination in some field of knowledge, undertaken to establish facts or principles; laborious or continued search after truth."[1] Gilbert A. Churchill, quoting the American Marketing Association, tells us that research is the "systematic gathering, recording, and analyzing of data about problems."[2] Churchill elaborates, pointing out that research emphasizes the **systematic** gathering of data; "one does not simply secure those data that are convenient or easily accessible." He continues, noting the implicit requirement that "the data are **objectively** and **accurately** gathered, recorded, and analyzed.[3] Implicit in both of these views is the notion that the research process should be careful, systematic, and objective.

Some rightly raise a tired objection: a human is a thinking, feeling being, with ideas and opinions, who has been brought up in a certain culture and time that he or she can never transcend. Therefore, it is quite impossible to be objective in conducting research. This argument is valid, but it quits too soon. It should go further, to argue that it is indeed good that we aren't objective, because our very lack of objectivity lends urgency and meaning to the quest for understanding of which research is a part. Researchers cannot be truly objective, but they can eliminate bias as much as possible from their work, and every effort should be made to be as careful and systematic as possible, and to avoid as much as possible introducing systematic bias into the assessment investigation.

Primary versus Secondary Research

Research can be grouped into two categories: secondary and primary. The nature of the research depends exclusively on the nature of the sources being consulted. Secondary research involves investigation of a question or problem, using only sources of information that have already been published. Some common secondary sources are census data, newspaper articles, letters and diaries, federal housing reports, and state hospital association discharge statistics. In contrast, primary research involves addressing a question or collecting information especially for the study at hand, usually by creating data that did not exist prior to the study. Generally, some sort of survey research, which we will discuss later, will be involved—either personal interviews, telephone interviews, mailed surveys, or a group interview process, which we will get into later.

The guides referred to in the chapter of models on community health needs assessments discuss a range of secondary data sources that will help you in locating and using secondary data, and some even provide whole rafts of data in the workbooks themselves. Help in conducting primary research is not forthcoming from these sources, however, so I will focus on conducting primary research.

Qualitative and Quantitative Research

Two types of primary research are qualitative and quantitative. Each is valid and offers much to researchers. Qualitative research focuses on, again quoting Webster, "that which belongs to something and makes or helps to make it what it is; characteristic element; attribute; as, purity of tone is an important quality of music."[4] A qualitative study investigates qualities, attributes, or characteristics. It probes and analyzes patterns of thought and preference. A qualitative study covers relatively few participants, to understand their thoughts and assumptions without regard to a larger audience. A study conducted to explore attributes that people associate with good physicians might serve as an example of a qualitative study. A qualitative study asks questions of how, when, where, why, and for what reason. The goal of the research is to understand the thoughts and feelings of the people themselves. Results from qualitative studies are generally reported in standard English.

In contrast, the concept of quantitative research has the concept of quantity embedded in it. As distinguished from qualitative research, the concept of quantitative research has to do with measurement. The quantitative study asks for quotations of how much, how big, and how often. A quantitative study will seek the responses of a relatively small sample of people, with the intent to generalize to a larger audience. Examples of quantitative studies would be (1) a study to measure the size of the market for a dialysis unit, as an example of a quantitative study, and (2) a survey of 400 households in your community in an effort to measure the use of hospital care. Results of quantitative studies are generally reported in percentages, correlation coefficients, indexes, and often in charts and graphs.

PRIMARY DATA COLLECTION METHODS

Ways to Conduct Primary Research

There are three ways, and only three ways, to conduct primary research: over the telephone, through the mail, or in person. These are tools only, and nothing about them is inherently "good" or "bad." Instead, each has specific attributes, which make them either useful or not useful, depending on a given situation. For example, shovels and flyswatters are tools. If you wanted to dig a ditch, you would use a shovel, not a flyswatter. If you wished to kill a fly, you would consider using a flyswatter, not a shovel. However, if the ditch you wish to dig is a very big ditch, you may wish to hire a contractor, who would use some sort of earth moving equipment; and if you wished to prepare your patio for a party, you may wish to fog the area, rather than use a flyswatter. Or, if you had a lot of flies to kill, you might want to investigate the reasons why there were so many flies in the first place. Maybe the trash can should be cleaned. Get the idea?

Later on, I discuss the research process, but for now I wish to discuss briefly some of the most frequently used research techniques. Let's think about a number of commonly used research techniques. If you have been paying attention during the past seven chapters, you will know I feel strongly that you should use a professional researcher to conduct your research. Such individuals have the experience, and will do a better job than you will. Many of you are rightly concerned about cost. Often researchers' fees seem expensive. However, if you were to determine all of the tasks and facilities required, then compare the real costs of doing the same quality of work yourself or of hiring an independent researcher to do it for you, you may find that hiring a reputable researcher will be less expensive. In addition, the researcher will do a better job, because he or she has the equipment and skills to do a first-rate job. I do not argue that you should be uninvolved in the work. However, your role should lie in working with the researcher to design the study, and then working to implement the results of the study. But if you decide to plunge ahead yourself, I present the following for you to think about in planning your work, and to give you guidance so you can avoid some basic errors. I have not been exhaustive; there are myriad details to consider.

TELEPHONE SURVEYS

What Is a Telephone Survey?

A telephone survey samples the opinions of people by using the telephone. An interviewer contacts one or more people, referred to as "respondents," by telephone and asks a list of questions, ranging from either a few to several hundred questions, according to a preestablished protocol. Respondents respond to each question, and, at the close of the interview, the interviewer thanks the respondent and hangs up. Questions may be designed for quantitative or qualitative research.

Telephone surveys are common in America today. Many of those who read this book have participated, or have refused to participate, in a telephone survey. Subjects appropriate for such surveys range from the type of soup people eat to their attitudes about sexual behavior. One finds them widely discussed with regard to political polls. Many political consultants earn a good living by conducting and interpreting the results of polls. Many politicians rely on them heavily to measure their success. Polls are bragged about when the results show a particular candidate doing well and are belittled by candidates shown to be "weak in the polls." Healthcare organizations often rely on telephone surveys as well.

The Interviewer and the Respondent

The central fact you should understand about a telephone survey is the not revolutionary idea that data are collected, after an interviewer calls a potential respondent and convinces that respondent to agree to answer a list of questions. Therefore, the quality of the answers given is affected by (1) the voice and demeanor of the interviewer, (2) whatever is going on at the place from which the interviewer is calling, (3) whatever is going on in the household that is called, and (4) whatever assumptions the respondent has about telemarketing and survey research. Before the interaction occurs, the interviewer does not know anything about the respondent, and the respondent is not aware the interviewer is going to contact him or her. From this central fact, several others inevitably follow. First, the respondent cannot see the interviewer or the way the interviewer is dressed or what the interviewer looks like. The visual context of the interview on the interviewer side does not come into play and does not affect the quality of the interview. And, because the interviewer cannot see the respondent, the way the respondent is dressed or looks does not affect the interviewer. But, because the two actors in this drama are shielded from each other, neither has very good information about the other.

Second, because the interviewer cannot know ahead of time what is going on in the respondent's household, the interviewer cannot be sure what the interviewer will find when the respondent is called. It may be during dinner; the respondent may have just have experienced a personal tragedy; the respondent may just have had a fight with another family member; the respondent may be watching his or her favorite television program; or a child may be pressuring the respondent to do something, such as attend a sporting event or take him or her shopping. The interviewer, therefore, must be very alert and sensitive to the constraints placed on the interview by such factors. Third, because the respondent doesn't know the nature of the questions, the interviewer may want the respondent to talk about things he or she hasn't spent a lot of time thinking about, may not know much about, or may not care much about. The voice and demeanor of the interviewer are paramount in securing the agreement of the participant to participate in the survey and to give accurate information. Finally, whatever is going on at the place from where the interviewer is calling is important. The quality of the data collected can be jeopardized if there is a lot of commotion behind the interviewer, if the interviewer is distracted, or if the interviewer has not been trained well on how to ask the questions. All of these "facts of life" may affect the quality of information achieved.

Completion Time

Telephone surveys can be completed within a matter of days or weeks. Some of our larger, better-known firms, with hundreds of interviewing positions across the country, conduct brief polls with thousands of respondents overnight. The data collection portion of a research study can be abbreviated simply by adding more interviewers to the telephone bank or by shortening the questionnaire. This can be a telling advantage if the study must be done in a short time.

Efficiency

Telephone interviews can be done efficiently. In the "good old days," telephone surveys were conducted using paper and pencil. As each interviewer conducted each interview, he or she filled checked boxes or wrote out responses on printed questionnaires, after which they were sent to an editor or staff of editors, who poured over each questionnaire to ensure that each was completed correctly. A coder then translated the responses on each edited questionnaire into a numeric coding scheme, then sent questionnaires to a data-entry operator, who entered the data into a computer file for analysis according to some preestablished criteria. In the "good *very* old days," the data-entry operator would have keypunched the responses onto a series of IBM cards to be read by a card reader or a computer. In those good *very* old days, completed and corrected questionnaires would have been sent to a research assistant, who would have counted responses manually and filled out data sheets that would be typed on a manual typewriter.

Today, we live in the world of the personal computer and the "information highway," and we can use computer-assisted telephone interviewing to make this system much more efficient. Today a questionnaire is developed and programmed on a computer. Interviewers sit at a terminal, call the respondents, and record the responses directly into a management data analysis system for manipulation and analysis. A computer-assisted telephone interviewing system yields more accurate data, because the software system prevents incorrect entries, eliminates coding and editing, and reduces the amount of time between the completion of the data collection and the analysis.

Of computers, there are two types: networked and stand-alone. Briefly, a networked system consists of a central computer, called a file server, and any number of "dumb" terminals, computerlike machines that can only function when connected to the file server. A stand-alone system functions on "smart" terminals, personal computers used as individual work stations when not involved in the research. The networked system has some distinct advantages over the stand-alone system, but the network versions are much more expensive to purchase and to operate. At my firm, we use the stand-alone system. We have debated purchasing the networked system but cannot convince ourselves that the advantages of the networked system are worth the additional investment. Most reputable firms today use a computer-assisted telephone system, either stand-alone or networked. Still, firms that use the paper and pencil method can produce high-quality data. You should not disqualify a firm that does not use a computer-assisted telephone interviewing system unless you find it deficient in some other way.

Flexibility

Telephone surveys are very flexible. The researcher can ask both structured and unstructured questions. Structured questions are most often used in quantitative research, as in "How satisfied were you with your last visit at Mount Saint Helen's Regional Hospital; would you say you were very satisfied, somewhat satisfied, somewhat unsatisfied, or very unsatisfied?" We can then create an average score and compare that score by certain user groups, and so forth. Unstructured questions are best suited in qualitative research, as in "How would you describe your most recent visit to Mount Saint Helen's Regional Medical Center?" We can review the words used in response to the question and then infer from that the basic attributes people ascribe to a positive patient encounter.

Probing and Clarifying

Telephone interviews offer the additional advantage of being able to probe respondents and clarify their responses. When probing a response, the interviewer asks for additional information. For example, an interviewer might ask, "What is the most pressing health need in your community?" The respondent might respond "lack of pediatric services." The interviewer might probe the respondent as follows: "What other problems does your community face?" The interviewer can continue this process until the respondent's thoughts are exhausted on the subject. In clarifying a response, the interviewer asks the respondent to elaborate or make clearer the meaning of the response. To clarify the response in the above example, an interviewer might ask, "How specifically is this a problem?"

This capability of probing and clarifying offers a further advantage of explanation. One may wish to explore an area that is not clear to very many respondents. For example, the health needs task force of Bobcat, Wyoming, located in the central part of the state, may wish to determine the degree to which people in central Wyoming would be receptive to establishing an HMO in the area. However, planners may be unsure about how familiar people in the community are with the concept of an HMO and may wish to measure the level of understanding of what an HMO is. An interviewer may ask the respondent, "How familiar are you with the term HMO?" Those who say they know what an HMO is can be asked to explain the term to the interviewer, and the interviewer can either write down the given explanations or judge in some way the degree to which a given explanation is accurate. To those respondents who say they are unfamiliar with the concept of an HMO, the interviewer can give an explanation of an HMO and then ask if the respondent had ever heard of it. This approach might be helpful to community health planners in addressing the health needs of the community.

Randomness

Conducting a telephone survey often involves selecting a sample for analysis and then generalizing the results to the population as a whole. For the generalization to be accurate, it is important that the sample typify the population—that it be random. Randomness is guaranteed when every element of the population from which the sample is drawn has an equal chance of being included in the sample. That is, nothing about the sample makes it atypical of the population as a whole. Sampling is vulnerable to sampling error. There are a number of ways to guard against sampling error that produce systematic biases in the sample, and there are thousands of textbooks that discuss randomness and ways to achieve it. We shall be content here to make the point that the telephone survey, based on samples of random numbers, offers the best way of achieving a random response. Also, telephone surveys can reach those who don't list their names in the telephone book through random number generation methodologies.

Intrusiveness

There's no way around it; telephone surveys are intrusive. I conduct studies using telephone surveys for many of my clients, and I conduct many interviews myself, so I hear firsthand the irritation of many who are called. In fact, hardly a week goes by when someone does not express to me the irritation of having been called by "some g—d—n telemarketer," just as he or she was sitting down to dinner after a trying day at work. Telephone surveys are done most often when people are most likely to be home—that is, evenings and weekends. The telephone interview is a very private contact, and the phone offers entrée into a household at vulnerable times. This fact underscores the necessity, discussed earlier in this section, for interviewers to be on their most courteous behavior.

Cost

Telephone surveys are the most cost-effective way of collecting primary data, but they can require a relatively large investment. Budgets being what they are, you may think that a phone survey is out of your price range. There are ways to minimize the investment needed, and a reputable research firm will work with clients to pare down so they can afford the study. I know, however, that even when an administrator tells me there is no budget for research, money can be found if the board of the hospital is sufficiently motivated to conduct the study.

Ease of Design

Questionnaires to be administered by telephone are relatively simple to design. Because only the interviewers see the questions, there is no necessity to professionally print them to make them look nice. As long as the questions are valid, asked in the correct order and in the right way, and are clear, nothing particularly beautiful needs to be designed.

Process

The telephone survey is conducted according to the following process: formulating the research question; identifying needed information; developing a questionnaire; testing the questionnaire; revising the questionnaire in light of the test; programming the questionnaire on a computer-assisted telephone interviewing system; developing the sample; fielding the questionnaire; tabulating the results; analyzing the results; presenting results; and preparing a research report.

Interest

Telephone interviewing can be interesting work. Interviewers find a lot of information they never knew before. Many find it intriguing to learn things that only they know, and often you "meet" some interesting people during an interview, even if for just a fleeting time, and even though the respondent remains only a voice to the interviewer.

Frustration

At the same time, interviewing by telephone is frustrating. Often hours will go by when no interviews can be completed because of too many refusals, nasty respondents, too many disconnected numbers, or because a high school basketball game that evening ensured that hardly anyone was at home in your community. Good interviewers will persevere, but the experience can still be daunting.

Some Tips

Before conducting a telephone survey, you should consider the following tips.

Tip 1. *Hire good interviewers and train them.* The effectiveness of research over the telephone depends on the extent to which interviewers are trained. Research firms invest a lot of time and money in hiring and training interviewers. Good interviewers come in all ages, genders, sizes, and shapes, from high school students to grandmothers. An effective inter-

---

Hypothetical Telephone Survey

Overview
Sylvania Memorial hospital is a 229-bed, county-owned facility located in Piedmont, Pennsylvania. Piedmont is a small community 25 miles outside Philadelphia. The hospital shares its market with several large hospitals in Philadelphia as well as with rural hospitals in surrounding counties.

The hospital has been regarded as a worthwhile community facility, but recently it has been compiling anecdotal evidence that the hospital is not as mindful of the community as it should be. Several board members have become concerned that the public position of the hospital has become eroded.

Objectives
- Identify the community's perceptions of the primary health needs of the community.
- Determine how consumers think Sylvania Memorial Hospital is meeting the health needs of the community.
- Measure consumers' satisfaction with the care provided at Sylvania Memorial Hospital.
- Measure the share of the market held by Sylvania Memorial Hospital relative to other area hospitals.
- Identify needed services and service gaps in Sylvania Memorial Hospital's service area.

Approach
The hospital commissioned a telephone survey of residents of Sylvania County and four communities outside the county: Ackland, Flat Spring, Skeltonville, and Mortontown. Interviews lasted from 10 to 15 minutes and were conducted with the heads of household sampled randomly from the hospital's service area, according to the proportion of households that each community contributed to the area as a whole.

The hospital also commissioned a survey of community leaders and social service agencies that served the community.

---

viewer must have a strong ego, be poised, unafraid of calling complete strangers over the phone, have a good telephone voice, communicate well over the telephone, be able to follow rather complicated instructions, and be adept at handling a variety of situations, some of which may be bizarre or even comical. In addition, the interviewers must be reliable enough to show up for work, be willing to ask questions if they are unsure of how to handle an unusual situation, and be willing to follow the instructions of the supervisor. I cannot stress highly enough the importance of training.

Tip 2. *Have interviewers call from a central location.* It is important for telephone interviews to be conducted from a central location. In the good old days, before the development of sophisticated and complex telephone equipment, research companies hired women (who used to be called "housewives") to conduct telephone interviews from their kitchen tables. Telephone supervisors used to drive from house to house, or be available by telephone, to answer questions and handle situations as they arose. This practice may still be used in some areas, but the industry has generally abandoned this practice in favor of central phone bank facilities. If you are thinking about doing your own telephone interviewing, I strongly recommend against having volunteers calling from their homes.

Tip 3. *Supervise interviewers carefully, continuously, and consistently.* Interviewing is often unpredictable, and interviewers must have a qualified person available to handle all the unforeseen events that may occur. Telephone interviewing at best can be routine, repetitive, and frustrating; but it can also be somewhat harrowing, especially if an interviewer encounters an abusive respondent. A few years ago, we were asking people in one area of Illinois about their health insurance. One evening, a new interviewer, on her first interview and during her first shift, called someone who told her emphatically and in no uncertain terms: "I don't want to take no f—ing survey." She fled in tears to the supervisor, who was able to calm her and assure her that this was very unusual. She had several very interesting interviews after that and turned out to be one of our best interviewers. Such unpleasant experiences characterize only the minority of contacts with respondents, but they can happen. I relate this anecdote only because I want to illustrate the challenges that interviewers face. Volunteers, motivated by the good feelings engendered by participating in the care of their friends and relatives in their local hospital, may quail before the challenge of asking the same questions over and over to strangers over the telephone, evening after evening. After a few nights of enthusiasm, volunteers usually find that other things are more important in their lives, and those supervising them must be adept at finding new volunteers to take their place, training them, and managing them.

Tip 4. *Keep the questionnaire simple.* The more complex the questionnaire, the more likely it is that interviewers will make mistakes, because they have to keep too many things in mind. If you are using a paper and pencil questionnaire, reduce the amount of page flipping or complicated branching.

Tip 5. *Ask questions in the right way.* They must be clear to the respondent, neutral in tone, and you should not ask respondents to answer two questions with one answer. No "have you stopped beating your wife?" type questions, please; and no "everyone in town likes Community Memorial Community Hospital, what do you think about Community Memorial Community Hospital?" One fact about telephone surveys is that the way the question is asked will influence the answer.

Tip 6. *Order your questions correctly.* The way a respondent answers a question will be affected by what came before. If you are not careful, you can introduce certain distortions into the results, distortions the researchers call "order effects," which undermine the validity of results. If you ask, for example, a series of questions about your hospital, then ask respondents what hospitals they have heard of, the awareness level of your hospital may be artificially high because you just asked them about yours. There are specific rotation procedures that professional research firms use to eliminate order effects.

Tip 7. *Keep the length of the questionnaire to a minimum.* There should be no unnecessary questions. Before developing the instrument, you should have developed a good idea of why you need the information you need. These decisions will determine the questions to be asked. Be ruthless in weeding out unnecessary questions. Eliminate all questions that would produce information "nice to know." Unless you have a clearly defensible reason for asking a question, don't include it on the survey. Have someone go over the questionnaire with you and ask, "Why are you asking that question?" If you can't come up with an answer that feels right to you, get rid of the question.

I cannot stress too strongly the impact of length. The longer the interview, the more interviewing hours it takes to complete a survey, the more labor-intensive it is, and the more resources it requires. We find that it generally takes at least five minutes on the phone before any worthwhile information can be generated. I find that at least 10 minutes are normally required, and interviews run sometimes to 15 minutes. Occasionally, interviews can last 20 minutes or more, but this is unusual, and normally not recommended, except under certain circumstances. Our experience is that, for every interviewing hour, about 35 minutes are spent on interviewer breaks, dialing numbers, experiencing refusals, identifying disconnected numbers, waiting for people to come to the phone, rescheduling interviews, and other such activities. So, about 2.5 10-minute surveys can be completed in an hour, but only about 0.8 20-minute interviews can be completed in an hour.

Using these parameters, administering a 10-minute interview to 100 people requires about 40 hours of work (100/2.5), or 10 people about 4 hours each. However, administering a study relying on a 20-minute survey to 1,000 people would require about 1,250 interviewing hours (1,000/0.8); 10 people will require about 125 interviewing hours each. These figures do not include time for training and supervision, nor do they include the cost of making the calls or for any long-distance calls required.

Tip 8. *Make your sample large enough so that your study will be worthwhile, but won't bust your budget.* If you are conducting a series of qualitative interviews with community leaders, 20 respondents may be sufficient. However, if you are conducting a quantitative study of households in your community, you may need to call 400 or more respondents. Most surveys of this type are based on 200 to 500 completed calls; but if an unusually rich data set is desired, you may wish to complete 1,000 to 1,500 interviews. There are two factors you need to weigh in making this decision: cost and analytical power. If you do not have the resources to conduct a large survey and you wish only a quick overview of your community, you may need as few as 100 or 200 interviews. If you have more resources and you wish a very in-depth analysis, you may wish to do 500 or more.

Tip 9. *Sample correctly.* If you are considering a random household survey, you will need to make sure that your sample meets the requirement for randomness. Generally, a sample is considered "random" if each and every element in the population that you are sampling has an equal chance of being included in the sample. This means if you are in Peoria, and you wish to conduct a household survey of Peoria County, the county in which the city of Peoria lies, you have to make sure that every household in the area you want to study has an equal chance of being included. If your sampling misses the south side, your data will not be adequate to describe what you want to know about the south side. If you want to learn about women, make sure your sample contains only women. There are a number of different sampling "strategies," including proportionate, straight random, stratified, sequential, and so on. Many research textbooks describe various sampling methods, and sampling is a rather esoteric and complicated domain. If you are unsure, you should consult a qualified researcher for advice. If you are conducting a qualitative study, your task may be easier. Generally, there are fewer people to sample from, and your task is to make sure that you have included all the people you want to interview.

Before you sample for a quantitative study, you will need to decide whether to use a "listed" sample or a sample of unlisted telephone numbers. Often, a list can be developed from the phone book fairly efficiently. Numbers can be taken directly from the book; but if you decide to go this way, you must realize that you will miss those whose numbers are unlisted. This will not be a problem for you unless the unlisted parties differ in any significant way from those whose numbers are listed. This difficulty can be circumvented if some sort of "+ n" method can be used, where the researcher adds a number, such as 9 or 1, to each number that is selected from the phone book, for a list of random telephone numbers. Another option is to purchase random phone numbers from a company that specializes in selling random samples to survey research centers, survey firms, or organizations or individuals that conduct survey research. These companies have invested significant resources in fine-tuning their samples, and buying a sample can be less expensive than creating your own sample. A third option is to use some sort of software program that lists random numbers or can generate them for you. Whatever route you take, the results will not be valid unless all the previous tips have been taken.

Tip 10. *Know beforehand how you are going to analyze the data.* The survey will collect a lot of information. You will need to know how you are going to analyze it. For years, such tabulations were done "by hand." The development of the personal computer and other electronic means has made such efforts obsolete, and I cannot recommend strongly enough against "hand-tabbing." The process is cumbersome, time-consuming, and fraught with error. Lots of software programs are available, from Lotus, to SPSS, SASS, STATPAC, and others that will handle the information cleanly, efficiently, effectively, and powerfully, and will display your data in a clear and accessible manner. Some have argued that they have employees who aren't doing anything else, anyway, and who can be put on this task. My response is that, if they have time to do this, they should either not be working there or doing something else.

Tip 11. *Consult a qualified researcher at a state or local university, a state department of health, or a private research firm.* Often they will provide limited assistance free or for a reduced fee. There are a host of other questions to be addressed. Only a qualified professional can help you with them: Should the study be blind, or should it be identified as being for your hospital? Should you offer some sort of premium for participants for participating? How many households should be contacted? What questions do I need to ask? and so forth.

Tip 12. *As a general rule, steer clear of using volunteers.* Some hospital managers, out of a well-intentioned though misguided effort to save money for their hospitals, yield to the temptation to use volunteers as researchers. Generally, before you decide to go this route, make sure you understand all the requirements of good telephone research. If a hospital has a very uniquely dedicated and capable cadre of volunteers, and a hospital staff trained and willing to supervise them, you may get away with using them. Volunteers may make good interviewers, but, more often, volunteers have neither the desire nor the training to be good phone interviewers. Many volunteers are motivated by the intense joy they experience in helping take care of friends, neighbors, and others in their community. Many of them don't have any qualifications, except their desire to serve. This is a wonderful thing, and volunteers can play a vital and important role in the life of the community hospital. However, not very many of them get a reward from calling strangers on the phone and asking series of questions over and over again for hours at a time. After a few nights, most volunteers find themselves more interested in being with their families, or in taking out the garbage. The hospital is then left with the need to recruit new volunteers. Before you decide to use volunteers, you should weigh the benefits carefully. You may wish to hire a professional researcher to train your staff in conducting telephone research.

MAILED SURVEYS

What Is a Mailed Survey?

A mailed survey involves developing a research questionnaire and sending it to potential recipients through the mail. Recipients read a series of questions and indicate their responses to them by checking boxes or circling numbers that are associated with each question. The respondent, after completing the questionnaire, places the questionnaire in a self-addressed envelope especially provided and mails the response back to the researchers. Mailed surveys are especially popular because of the ease with which they can be carried out. Much of the work can be done in-house, and its structured format makes responses easy to tabulate and analyze.

Process

A mailed survey is conducted using the following process: formulating the research question; determining information needed to answer the question; developing the questionnaire; testing the questionnaire; revising the questionnaire, in light of the test; laying out and printing the questionnaire; coding the questionnaire; stuffing and mailing the questionnaire, together with a carefully worded cover letter, a stamped and self-addressed envelope, and an incentive, if used (more about that later); receiving the returned questionnaires; sending out a reminder card or second mailing; preparing questionnaires for data entry; entering the questionnaires into a data analysis software system; tabulating the responses; editing the data; analyzing the data; presenting the results; and preparing a research report.

Facts about Mailed Surveys

The central fact of mailed surveys is that the only mechanism affecting the interaction between researcher and respondent is a piece of mail. Other facts follow from this. First, only when the questionnaire arrives and how it looks when it arrives can encourage response. This means that you must take greater care in developing the questionnaire so it looks "nice," and that you must spend more time with the format of the questionnaire, typing envelopes, printing and stuffing, and that sort of thing. Second, it means there must be an accurate mailing list so you can get an accurate "read" of what the community thinks or does. Third, it also means the respondent can take more care with the questionnaire and think more about the subject of the study. Fourth, it means that the topics of the questionnaire must be clear to respondents, because no one will be available to explain things that aren't known clearly to the recipient. Fifth, it means that the researcher cannot probe and clarify effectively.

Investment

Mailed surveys are generally less expensive than telephone surveys. This is particularly true when a large-scale survey is planned. But for small-scale studies, mailed surveys may be more expensive, because administrative costs are higher—that is, more money is spent for printing, postage, and other clerical costs.

Intrusiveness

A mailed questionnaire is the least intrusive research technique and is often recommended when the subject matter of a survey is rather sensitive or when some thought on the part of respondents is desirable.

Hypothetical Mailed Survey

Overview
A Wisconsin-based health maintenance organization wished to evaluate the quality of the service that its affiliated hospitals provided its members. The HMO's management had recently commissioned a series of focus groups to identify the key determinants of member satisfaction. The HMO then wished to conduct a mailed survey to measure the extent to which the results of the focus groups could be generalized to all members, and to evaluate the quality of service the members were receiving.

Approach
The HMO contacted a research firm, which assisted it in developing and implementing a mailed survey sent to 1,200 HMO members. The consultant helped the HMO management to develop the questions and consulted on layout and questionnaire design. The HMO formatted and printed the questionnaire internally, and its staff sent out the questionnaires to be returned directly to the research firm. The research firm tabulated the responses, analyzed the information, and presented results to the HMO's management.

Format

Mailed surveys work best when they are highly structured. They work worst when a lot of unstructured input is required. For example, in conducting a telephone survey, one can probe and clarify responses that are either unclear or somewhat off the mark. We discussed probing and clarifying earlier. If a respondent says your hospital stinks, the interviewer can ask the respondent to elaborate or be more specific. On a questionnaire filled out at home, if a respondent has written that your hospital stinks, you are stuck. If much unstructured input is required, you would be best to choose another research method.

Mailed surveys do not work well when branching is desired—that is, the researcher may wish to ask a special group of questions to respondents who fit specific criteria. For example, one may want to know what people who have used your hospital thought about various aspects of your hospital's service, and may wish to have everyone who did not use the hospital in the past year to skip that question. This offers no problems on a telephone survey where the interviewer controls the interaction with the respondent. However, using a mailed approach, the researcher will have to provide a set of instructions, or shade an area of the questionnaire, or draw an arrow, or do something else to tell the respondent to skip to another question. This creates confusion among respondents and may produce inaccurate information or unusable questionnaires.

Tips on Conducting a Mailed Questionnaire

Eleven come to mind. They are:

Tip 1. *Do not ask about topics that are not widely known.* Make sure the topic is very clear and well understood by potential recipients. If the topic is vague, not well understood, or requires extensive explanation, the odds of success are considerably less.

Tip 2. *Format with care.* Take special care to lay out and format questionnaires clearly and attractively. We used to rely on professional printing companies to handle this; these days, a number of desktop publishing systems can do it for you.

Tip 3. *Make questions structured.* Be sure questions are clear and structured, giving respondents easy ways to check boxes or circle numbers to indicate their responses. The success of a mailed survey hinges on achieving as high a response rate as possible from as representative a cross-section of the target population as possible.

Tip 4. *Weed out unnecessary questions.* Ask only questions that collect information you absolutely need, and have a good idea of why you are asking each question, as in the previous section on telephone surveys.

Tip 5. *Avoid open-ended questions.* Use such questions as infrequently as possible. They generally produce information that can't be used.

Tip 6. *Avoid branching as much as possible.* In conducting telephone surveys, we often "branch" questions—that is, we often ask a series of questions to respondents who answer a previous question in a given way. For example, we may ask respondents, "Please name all the hospitals you have heard of in your area"; and then, "What word or phrase comes to mind when you think of (hospital name)?" for each hospital they mention. Those that didn't mention a given hospital are skipped along to a subsequent question. This approach is generally less successful in mailed surveys, because people often misread the instructions and skip to the wrong place in the questionnaire.

Tip 7. *Make sure you have a valid mailing list.* One of my earliest projects foundered because, during the test, the huge number of undelivered mailings that were returned told us that the mailing list was old and inaccurate. The project was suspended, and the funds budgeted for it were shifted to purchase new software to update the mailing list. The client didn't find out the information he said he wanted, but he did improve his mailing list.

Tip 8. *Take scrupulous care in layout and design.* Lay out and design the appearance of the questionnaire carefully. Because there is no interviewer to encourage responses, the questionnaire must be attractive and easy to read, and the questions need to be clear and concise.

Tip 9. *Include with the questionnaire a cover letter and a stamped self-addressed envelope.* Make sure you include in each mailing a carefully drafted cover letter, plus a stamped and self-addressed envelope. Envelopes should be personalized as much as possible, and bulk mailings should be avoided. If at all possible, have addresses typed directly on the envelope, avoiding mailing labels altogether.

Tip 10. *Notify and remind.* You should follow up each mailing with a reminder post card or a second mailing about a week after the initial mailing. A notification card should be sent about a week before the initial mailing.

Tip 11. *Plan for the questionnaire to arrive in the middle of the week.* Plan for the questionnaire to arrive at its destination on Tuesday, Wednesday, or Thursday. Monday is the heaviest mail day; and if your mailing arrives on Monday, chances are greater that your piece will be ignored or thrown out. On Friday, people are thinking about the weekend, and chances are greater that it will find itself on the bottom of a pile of mail or in the wastebasket.

FOCUS GROUPS

A focus group comprises six to 12 people, carefully recruited, who engage in a carefully planned and organized discussion led by a skilled moderator who "focuses" the discussion on a topic or group of related topics that are of interest to the sponsor by asking a number of carefully crafted questions in a specifically determined order. The technique has been adapted, with some violence done to it, from psychiatric therapy models, wherein the therapist tries to tap the "unconscious" mind of patients through interaction with other patients. Fortunately, the technique has proved robust enough to weather its transplant from therapy to research. The focus group is unique, because it offers the sponsor of the focus group the opportunity to observe participants and hear what they say from their own lips, unscarred by glib market research jargon. Often what the participants say is quite remarkable and often unanticipated by those watching the group. But, whether what one hears is a revelation or an irrelevancy is always problematic. Unfortunately, though the technique requires very careful preparation and implementation, the term *focus group* has become so widely used that it has been trendily snatched by those unqualified to use it, under the guise of having done "in-house research."

Often people say "focus group" when they refer indiscriminately to some informal feedback session with participants. There is nothing wrong with feedback sessions, open-houses, town meetings, and the like. They are very valuable and should be done. My quarrel is that they are passed off as focus groups when they aren't, thereby increasing the amount of misinformation about real focus groups.

Process

Conducting a focus group study involves the following steps: (1) formulating the research question; (2) determining the information needed; (3) determining the characteristics of participants to be recruited; (4) determining the number of groups to be held; (5) arranging for a facility and for any specialized equipment you will need, such as videotaping equipment, VCR, and so on; (6) scheduling the groups; (7) recruiting the participants; (8) designing the focus group script, which details the questions to be asked, probes to be used, and the order in which they will be asked; (9) notifying participants by mail; (10) reminding the participants on the day or the night before the group meeting; (11) moderating the groups; (12) writing the summary; and (13) presenting the results.

Facts about Focus Groups

The central facts defining a focus group are these: (1) people are in a room together; (2) a skilled moderator leads the group; (3) questions are carefully crafted; and (4) the situation they are in is artificial. Several other facts flow from these. A key characteristic of the focus group is the presence of everyone in a room—they can all see each other. The quality of the information is affected by the way people are dressed and behave; the way the moderator dresses and behaves; the kind of room; and temperature, sounds, atmosphere, and other such environmental attributes. If one person in the group is allowed to "grandstand," it will silence everyone else. If a prominent person is "in" with others, the information will be distorted. Second, people are selected carefully. Carefully designed recruitment procedures should be used to ensure that the right kind of respondents are recruited for the study, and rigorous procedures that are designed to encourage participation must be in place. Third, people in the room are encouraged to bring up and discuss thoughts and ideas they hadn't thought of before. In fact, the most exciting focus groups are those in which the group takes on a life of its own and people share their thoughts and feelings about an issue or product. This can be good if the information "learned" really guides one to thoughts and feelings that define the way they actually think. However, it can be dangerous, if they are "off on a tangent," in a way that only seems insightful but is really quite irrelevant. Sometimes, it is hard to know which. Fourth, these interactions among the participants take place in an artificial situation. The decor of the room in which they are held, the height and comfort of the chairs, the time, and any exogenous events like high school basketball tournaments, Monday Night Football, or a school concert—all can affect the outcome of the group. This artificiality often can free people's minds to speak openly, but it means that people aren't as comfortable as they would be at home, and they often are somewhat disoriented by having to leave home, get a ride, and find their way to an unfamiliar location. Also, many are suspicious that the focus group may in fact be a disguised sales pitch. Fifth, the focus group's results cannot be generalized to the population as a whole. They are and always will remain the product of that particular group of people at that particular time. One cannot say that, because half of the people of the focus group thought a given way, half of the community thought a given way. In fact, a focus group remains one data point, even if there are 12 people in the group, and one can only generalize about what participants in one focus group said, compared with what participants in other focus groups said. Sixth is the presence of the moderator. The moderator is key to a successful focus group. The moderator's skill at dealing with dominant people in the group, encouraging silent people to speak, following up some ideas but not others, putting people at ease, and dealing with the thousand other issues arising unpredictably in a group will determine the success of the group.

Focus Groups at Their Best

Focus groups are at their best when the topics chosen are conceptually fuzzy, or when the items asked about must be seen, heard, felt, or tasted. I have used focus groups for taste tests; I have shown participants television advertisements; I have presented them with newsletters and printed advertising copy; and I have confronted participants with any number of usual or somewhat unusual items. Focus groups are never predictable; anything can happen and usually does.

Flexibility

Focus groups can be conducted in any setting that is appropriate to the study. Potential locations include people's homes, hotel rooms, public libraries, community centers, restaurant facilities, or professional focus group facilities. Many are conducted in professional focus group facilities. Such facilities are convenient for the moderator, because they are designed to handle focus groups and therefore are staffed and specially equipped with client viewing rooms, one-way mirrors, hidden microphones, videotaping equipment, televisions, VCRs, refrigerators, ovens, and all sorts of utensils, pots and pans, cups, and plates, thereby able to handle focus groups efficiently and easily.

A professional focus group facility is not required, however. Successful focus groups can be conducted in any meeting room that is accessible and appropriate. I have conducted groups in professional facilities; but I have also conducted them in public libraries, restaurant meeting rooms, and hotel conference centers. One of my most successful groups was held in a small room in a bar in a very small town in southeastern Minnesota; one of my least successful groups was held in a fancy focus group facility in Kansas City, Missouri. Often, these other locations are cheaper, and sometimes you can get them for free if you know the right people. It is generally recommended not to hold focus groups in your hospital's meeting room, but this depends on the situation.

Completion Time

Focus groups can be conducted quickly, sometimes in a matter of a few weeks, from start to finish. They are flexible. They can be used in almost any situation and under almost any conditions. They are especially good for exploratory research, because they offer a window into the way people think and feel, and they provide a forum in which one person's responses will spark responses of others.

Special Handling

The characteristics of the population under study require special handling. If the researcher wants to probe how well the hospital is meeting the needs of recently discharged cancer patients or patients seriously ill with diabetes, the project may founder on the inability of patients to get around

---

Hypothetical Focus Group

Overview
A Local Community, Ohio, task force was considering the feasibility of establishing a low-cost, community-based clinic designed to improve medical care for adolescents. Local Community Hospital, a 154-bed facility, was interested in providing facilities for the clinic as a way of addressing a perceived need in the community. A local foundation had expressed interest in providing startup funds for the project. To evaluate the feasibility of establishing such a clinic, and to understand the features that such a center should incorporate, the task force contracted with a local moderator to conduct a series of focus groups with teenagers and parents of teenagers.

Objectives
  • To describe the conditions under which teenagers would be most likely to use the clinic.
  • To explore the perceptions of teens concerning medical services.
  • To probe teenagers' response to the concept of a low-cost, community-based clinic for teenagers.
  • To investigate teenagers' reactions to potential service attributes.

Approach
The moderator met with the task force to identify the information needed, establish recruiting criteria, determine the number of groups needed, and establish other protocols to guide the research.

---

easily. Some groups require special treatment. Physicians, for example, tend to "grandstand," unless held in check by an experienced moderator. In addition, paying a physician to participate in a focus group may run up to $200 per physician, especially if he or she is a specialist, such as an anesthesiologist, who places a high monetary value on time. I usually recommend against focus groups with physicians, in favor of personal interviewing.

Tips on Conducting a Focus Group

Ten should do the trick.

Tip 1. *Make sure what you want to know.* Before you start, know what you want to know about, why you want to know about it, and how you are going to use the information afterward. If you know these things beforehand, the group's value to you will be enhanced. If you have not thought of these things, you are running against a current of irrelevancy.

Tip 2. *Have a clear idea of whom you want to know about.* Know the types of people you wish to have in the group. Specify quotas if necessary, such as four people aged 18 to 34; four people aged 35 to 54; and four people over the age of 55; or all women, half under 50 and half over 50.

Tip 3. *Hire good interviewers to recruit participants.* Those who recruit participants need to have a brief survey, so they can recruit the needed individuals. You should follow the same tips regarding interviewers as noted in the section under telephone interviewing tips.

Tip 4. *Allow enough time for recruitment and notification.* For people to attend the group, they have to know when the meeting is to be held, where, and how to get there. Be sure to send a letter to each participant about one week ahead of time, with a map, and contact those who have agreed to participate either the night before or the day of the focus group to remind them.

Tip 5. *Pay participants a reasonable sum.* It is only fair to the participants to reimburse them for their time and expense in attending your group. It also encourages participation. There is nothing more frustrating than trying to hold a group in which only one or two or perhaps no participants come. The amount to be paid should vary according to the participant. We generally pay consumers, depending on location and the type of individual involved, $35 to $50 per participant. If you are contemplating a focus group with physicians, we recommend paying, depending on specialty, $100 to $200 per physician. Paying in cash at the conclusion of the group is best.

Tip 6. *Consult a professional for training in conducting a focus group.* Often a professional will spend some time with you discussing focus group techniques. Not everyone can be a good moderator; and if you have had no experience in these matters, you may wish to use an independent moderator.

Tip 7. *Conduct the group outside your institution.* If the focus group is to be a blind study, you will need an outside site to protect the identity of the sponsor. If it is not a blind group, you will find a more open audience if you are not sitting in the hospital itself. As I noted above, a meeting room in the local public library might work quite well, and for a very reasonable fee. Make sure that the room is clean, comfortable, and homey.

Tip 8. *Provide refreshments.* If the group is to be held around dinner time, you may wish to serve dinner in conjunction with the group. If not, you should have on hand some light snacks, coffee, juices, soft drinks, fruit, rolls, or anything else appropriate. Be sure to have decaffeinated beverages and low-fat food available.

Tip 9. *Have someone help you.* There are a number of things to do, such as greeting people, checking off attendance lists, and so on. That way, you can concentrate on greeting the people, making them feel at home, and conducting the group. A helper handles details.

Tip 10. *Tape the group.* Make sure you have a good microphone that will cover the area of the room. Models are available commercially that do not look like microphones and work well. Make sure you tell people you are taping their comments. They will figure it out, anyway, and you should communicate to them the fact that the effort is on the up and up. You will want to refer to the tapes later to clarify some points, or allow others to listen to the group.

PERSONAL INTERVIEWING

Personal interviewing can be very useful. For interviewing physicians, business leaders, or other busy people who have limited time, interviewing them in their offices is recommended. This normally consists of an interviewer matched one-on-one with an interviewee, though in some situations two or three people may be interviewed concurrently. The process of conducting personal interviews is similar to conducting telephone interviews. Personal interviews can be used most cost-effectively to elicit in-depth information, often rather sensitive, on a relatively small number of people, say 25 or fewer. Personal interviewing can be done over the telephone or in person. Conducted over the telephone, personal interviewing may not be very different from a small-scale telephone interview, except that the interviewer is generally more skilled at interviewing; the interviewee is usually a leader in the community or a professional field, such as a corporation executive, a physician, or the CEO of a hospital; and the interview is generally more unstructured and qualitative in nature.

Personal interviews conducted in person can require a substantial investment, if those to be interviewed are spread across the country or internationally. It becomes expensive to fly one researcher around to different parts of the country, and added cost can be incurred if the interviewee cancels the appointment and must be rescheduled. In such cases, it often works well to hire trained interviewers in the communities themselves, though this practice may jeopardize inter-interviewer reliability. Interviewing people in your community in person, however, usually is not prone to such difficulties.

An important feature of a personal interview conducted in person is the fact that the interviewer and the respondent are in the same room. Hence, how the interviewer looks and acts, how the interviewer behaves, and how he or she talks have a strong impact on the quality of the interview.

Tips on Conducting a Personal Interview

Follow these tips for a successful personal interview:

Tip 1. *If possible, use an independent interviewer.* Respondents may not feel comfortable sharing their most inner thoughts with you, but they may be more open to a stranger. Clients have often told me that they have heard people they knew say things to me they never heard from them themselves. The interviewer may also be more experienced at interviewing than you are.

Tip 2. *Allow extra time for making appointments.* Remember that people you are trying to reach are busy, and it may require several phone calls to set up an appointment.

Tip 3. *Build in time to reschedule interviews.* I have not yet conducted a study in which everyone I was to interview was available when they said they would be. Many of them are busy, and things come up that demand their attention. Others really don't want to talk to you, but don't like to say so, and, instead, cancel without warning. The person to be interviewed may not be available at the time the initial appointment was made.

OTHER DATA COLLECTION METHODS

Mall Intercepts

A mall intercept involves approaching people in a shopping mall or other centralized public location and asking them either to participate in a personal interview or fill out a self-administered questionnaire. Mall intercepts are popular because they are handy. Many research companies have offices in malls so they can complete these kinds of surveys. This approach can be helpful for exploratory research. But for important studies, they should be handled carefully and should be avoided unless the precise characteristics of desired participants are known and respondents can be qualified carefully to make sure they fit the desired characteristics.

Here are some tips for conducting a mall intercept:

Tip 1. *Make sure you use the right mall.* If you wish to find out about the preferences or thoughts of low-income residents of your community, select a mall they often use. It will do little for you if you select a mall in a high-income area.

Tip 2. *Make sure you can get access to the mall you wish to use.* Many malls do not allow research at all. Others allow it, but have an exclusive contract with a professional market research firm. Others allow research to be conducted and do not have an exclusive contract, but charge very high fees.

Tip 3. *Know the type of people you wish to interview.* It is unlikely that the sample of people you speak with in a mall will be random. Malls are located in places. This means that a mall will attract people in inverse proportion to the distance between their residence and the mall. Have specific quotas for people, and qualify people in the mall carefully to make sure you are getting the right mix of respondents.

Tip 4. *Learn as much as you can about the mall the day you want to use it.* Know what will be happening in the mall during the time you wish to be there. Malls are designed to sell goods and services. By researching people in malls, you are only surveying those who spend more time shopping, and special sales in malls draw a disproportionate share of some people over others. You will not necessarily know what sales will be on when you plan your study. To make money, malls often allow groups to display special wares in the concourses, such as cars, jewelry, real estate photos, or other items, and they promote these heavily. This will attract a disproportionate share of people to the mall. You may not know exactly what group is going to be showing until the day you go to the mall for the research.

Tip 5. *Make sure you cover all entrances.* Malls have many of them, and, unless interviewers are placed strategically to ensure even coverage, your sample may not be random.

Tip 6. *Woo mall managers.* Most managers are dedicated to making money for the corporation that owns the mall. This is their job, they do it very well, and they should be complimented. Most mall managers guard carefully against researchers, because they are afraid that the presence of researchers will scare off shoppers and reduce sales. If you know someone who runs a local mall, and the mall is located in the right area, and the mall owner is a community-minded person, he or she may allow you to use the mall at no charge or a reduced fee. But be sure that the management will not place any restrictions on you that will jeopardize your project.

Door-to-Door Surveys

These surveys were used frequently long ago when people were home during the day and when neighborhoods were perceived as safe. They involved a personal interview conducted by researchers who combed a neighborhood and interviewed people in each residence. These are still done occasionally; however, the development of more sophisticated technology and equipment, the decline of the traditional family, and growing concerns about safety, both for the interviewer and the interviewee, have reduced the desirability of this kind of research. There is a further serious methodological challenge to guarantee that the sample of interviewees will be random.

Lobby Surveys

This survey is a kind of exit poll, carried out in the lobby of a hospital, bank, or other place where people congregate. For example, researchers may wish to measure the satisfaction of people with the appointment desk at the local hospital by interviewing people as they leave the hospital. These surveys can be very useful, because it will be relatively easy to find people to complete the project, and those in the lobby or waiting area will be those whom you would wish to survey. The researcher should keep in mind that the research will apply only to those people who visited the hospital on that day at that time, so you should consider carefully the days of the week and the times of the day the interviewing is carried out. Further, hospitals, like malls, have many different entrances. The research design should also take this into consideration and place interviewers strategically. For example, an evaluation of emergency room patients may not be done effectively if interviewers are not placed near the emergency room exit.

Hybrid Approaches

Researchers have a large number of research methods to choose from. In addition to the ones outlined above, researchers can mail things to people, then call them and interview them. They can ask a sample of people to watch a given advertisement at home, then either send them a written survey or interview them by telephone. Researchers in a mall can qualify shoppers and recruit them for an in-depth interview at a different time and location. One can arrange to display a product or service in a mall on a Saturday afternoon, and then interview people who visited the display.

Researchers can invite employees to a meeting and administer a survey to them in an "in-class" setting. Any research method will be appropriate as long as it enables the researchers to answer the questions they have formulated, the method will work, and the researchers have the resources to carry it out. Before selecting a method, you should consult a qualified independent research professional.

Future Trends

Rapid changes in computer hardware and software and in communication technology is breaking down the barriers between the researchers and respondents. One impact may be that the telephone survey and the personal interview may not be very different. As I see it, there are at least four trends.

Trend 1. *The telephone interviewer will be able to see the respondent.* Much of the advantages of personal interviewing will accrue to the telephone survey, and interviewing people in person will become less advantageous. The respondent will be able to see the interviewer as well, so what the interviewer wears, what he or she looks like, and the background of the interviewer will now affect the quality of the interview.

Trend 2. *The telephone interviewer will be able to show things to the respondent and ask questions about them.* It is not implausible to think that, in the not too distant future, researchers will actually be able to play a videotape of an advertisement or other message on the respondent's television set and get immediate feedback. It used to be possible to do this only in a focus group.

Trend 3. *Focus groups will be conducted differently.* It used to be necessary, and still is necessary in most cases, for moderators, sponsors, and participants alike to physically travel to a central location to conduct the groups. Not so, down the road. It will be possible, and now is sometimes possible, for people in very remote locations to be plugged into a video conference and participate with each other and talk to each other as though they were in the same room. As virtual reality software becomes better and more common, it may also be possible for people separated by hundreds of miles to actually touch, feel, and experience items and give their immediate feedback.

Trend 4. *Changes in statistical analysis software may make it easier for surveys to be tabulated and analyzed.* For several years we have had optical scanners, which can score mailed surveys, and future scanners will be even quicker and more powerful. This means that mailed surveys and self-administered surveys will be more effective. In the future, it may be possible in many settings for the respondent to fill out a "mailed" questionnaire interactively via a computer screen. High-speed fax machines will drastically cut response time in some settings. Some "mailed" questionnaires may be completed and returned in a matter of minutes.

CONCLUSION

In review, my purpose in discussing research at this point is not to present a textbook on research methods. Shelves of books in the libraries of many universities discuss the topic comprehensively. Rather, the point of this discussion is merely to give you a sampling of information concerning various research techniques and what is involved in doing them well. Many details I have not covered and could only cover in relation to a given research project. I repeat my plea that you use a professional researcher to conduct your research for you, or that you at least consult a researcher as you are planning your study.

Should You Do Primary Research?

As I hope you can see from the material in this chapter, collecting primary research is a complicated affair. Whether you should depends on how you answer the two questions below. If you answer either one yes, you should start planning to collect some primary data.

1. Is the secondary information available to you out of date, unreliable, not specific to your community, or not credible for some other reason? _____

   _____

   _____

2. Is there a specific request for primary research from your hospital staff or from elsewhere in your community? _____

   _____

   _____

Should You Involve an Outside Firm?

By this time, you know my answer to this question. To find out yours, take this little test. Check the appropriate space next to each question. If you answer no to any one of these questions, you should involve an outside research firm, organization, or individual to help with at least some of it.

1. Do you have the expertise?
2. Do you have the budget?
3. Do you have the facilities?
4. Do you have the staff?
5. Do you have the time?

How to Know a Good Outside Firm When You See One

A good consultant will have the following attributes:

1. He or she will have been in the business for at least five years.
2. He or she will be knowledgable about some aspect of the health-care industry and be aware of recent changes.
3. Fees charged will be reasonable.
4. The consultant will have sound references.
5. The consultant will have had experience with assignments that are of comparable complexity; but past assignments may not necessarily be identical to the assignment he or she would pursue with you.
6. The consultant is skilled in conducting research but is not necessarily with a big-name firm. Face it, some of the best-known firms will not serve you the best. They will be more interested in collecting data that will maintain their reputation than they will be in working closely with you.
7. The consultant will consider doing things your way, to "unbundle" his or her consulting services to meet your wishes, as long as what you are asking him or her does not jeopardize the quality of research.
8. The consultant will return your calls promptly; on the same day if possible, but not later than the next day.
9. The consultant will respond with a proposal within a week, unless he or she is on vacation, in which case you should make exceptions.
10. The consultant will produce reports the way you want to see them, and on a schedule consistent with your requirements.
11. The consultant will be someone you would be comfortable taking to lunch with your best friend.
12. The consultant will have good writing and speaking skills, and have good grammar and spelling.

How to Handle a Consultant

If you engage a consultant, you should act in the following ways toward him or her. After all, consultants are people, too. Often clients expect certain behaviors from the consultant that they do not expect of themselves.

1. If you ask a consultant to prepare a proposal for you, put your ideas down in writing for him or her, even if you don't have an official "request for proposal" to issue.

2. Respond quickly to the proposal. Let the consultant know that you have received the proposal, and offer any immediate thoughts about the proposal if you have had a chance to review it.

3. If the consultant calls you, return his or her call promptly, even though you may have no news to report. If I had a nickel for every unreturned phone call, I would be very rich.

4. If a few weeks go by, and you have not made a decision, let the consultant know where he or she stands. Consultants invest a good deal of time, energy, money, and ego in their proposals, and it is very discouraging to hear nothing from potential clients, or to have phone calls go unreturned.

5. If you are unclear about anything related to the proposal, ask the consultant to clarify. You may have forgotten to tell the consultant something that he or she needed to know. If there is something else you may wish from the consultant, but couldn't find it in the proposal, ask about it.

6. If you turn down a proposal from a consultant, give the consultant specific feedback about the reasons why his or her proposal was not selected and what, if anything, the consultant could have done to have a better proposal. I am always looking for ways to improve, and I always learn more from proposals that are not accepted than from those that are accepted.

7. Make sure you agree on the fees early and take responsibility to ensure that the consultant's bills are paid in a timely fashion. Most of us expect that a check processing delay of about two to three weeks is normal and are pleased when we are paid faster.

8. Remember that consultants are under pressure, too. If your decisions are delayed, keep in mind that their work can't necessarily be speeded up. Try to remember that you and the consultant are on a team, and try to work together as colleagues.

ENDNOTES

1. *Webster's New Twentieth Century Dictionary of the English Language, Unabridged.* Edited by Jean L. McKechnie. Cleveland: World Publishing Company, 2d ed. 1963, pp. 1538–1539.

2. Churchill, Gilbert A. *Marketing Research: Methodological Foundations.* 3d ed. Hinsdale, IL: Dryden Press, 1983, p. 11.

3. Churchill, *Marketing Research*, p. 11.

4. Webster, p. 1474.

Chapter Ten

Statewide Survey

INTRODUCTION

This chapter trips you through sovereign territories, the landscape of community health needs assessments in America. We will be going fast. The areas through which we will be traveling will be undulating and changing before our eyes, and spokespersons with state hospital associations will act as our guides. Because the terrain is so volatile, this is not the only possible tour. And we won't stop at every state, because I couldn't get any information from some state associations. So, hold on. The tour is starting.

STATE HOSPITAL ASSOCIATIONS

Alabama

There is activity in Alabama, but it is not clear how much. The hospital association has not taken on community health assessment as a formal project. The hospital has pulled together some health statistics from the department of health and hopes to develop a data resource for hospitals seeking health statistics, but it has not produced specific products for its hospitals. Rather, it wishes to serve as a resource for local hospitals that are seeking assistance. There is no legislative mandate for community health needs assessments in Alabama, and, at present, there is no move to make it happen.

For more information, contact Ms. Rosemarie Blackmon, vice president for Public Relations and Membership, Alabama Hospital Association, 500 North East Blvd, Montgomery, Alabama 36117. Call (205) 272-8781.

Alaska

Virtually every community in Alaska is working to assess and improve its health status. There is no legislative mandate for it, but communities have plugged into the need of increased access and cost reduction. Alaska has three healthcare systems: (1) the federal health system encompassing native, military, and veterans hospitals; (2) the state system of nursing homes, psychiatric hospitals, and centers for developmentally disabled; and (3) the community hospital system, including both proprietary and nonproprietary. Sometimes a hospital initiates the process; sometimes other organizations initiate the process. The state association does not provide any consulting services, but it tries to facilitate the process whenever a hospital approaches it. When a hospital decides it wants to do community assessment, the association draws on one or more of four primary resources: AHA project, the healthcare forum's program for a healthier community, assistance from the Foundation for the Washington State Hospital Association, and the University of Washington School of Medicine. The challenge has been to coordinate and correlate and help those communities. If necessary, it will set up conference calls between communities and those with the resources to assist them.

For more information, contact Mr. Harlan Knudson, president, Alaska State Hospital and Nursing Home Association, 319 Seward Street, Suite 11, Juneau, Alaska. Call (907) 586-1790.

Arizona

I couldn't find much activity in Arizona. A few years ago, the Flynn Foundation financed a study that concentrated on rural health. The hospital association is looking at a range of projects in relation to community health needs assessments but has not identified a direction yet.

For more information, contact Ms. Bridget O'Gara, vice president of Communications, Arizona Hospital Association, 1501 W. Fountainhead Parkway, Suite 650, Tempe, Arizona 85282. Call (602) 968-1083.

Arkansas

There appears to be some interest in community health needs assessments among some hospitals, but, as far as the hospital association is aware, only a very few are interested. The hospital association has not developed a program for its hospitals but may do so in the future.

For more information, contact Mr. Paul Cunningham, vice president, Arkansas Hospital Association, 419 Natural Resources Drive, Little Rock, Arkansas 72205-1539. Call (501) 224-7878.

California

Recent legislation, flowing from a belief that hospitals are not worthy of their tax-exempt status, requires most community hospitals to conduct community health needs assessments and to submit community benefit plans to the state, beginning in 1997. Many hospitals were already involved in community health needs assessments, and, therefore, only had to put down in writing what they were already doing. Most of the activity seems to be coordinated through the hospital councils and the Catholic Hospital Association. The California Association of Hospitals and Health Systems does not provide technical assistance to hospitals. Rather, it prefers to facilitate the process and refers them to a consultant or to one of the councils. The association is developing an on-line computer program through which hospitals can talk to each other and gather information from each other. The association is also developing a library that hospitals can use in their search for information and resources.

For further information, contact Ms. Dorel Harms, vice president of Professional Services, California Association of Hospitals and Health Systems, 1201 K. Street, Suite 800, Sacramento, CA 95812. Call (916) 443-7401.

Colorado

A lot of activity exists in Colorado, particularly through the Colorado Action for Healthy People and the Colorado Partnership for Healthy Communities, in conjunction with the National Civic League. The hospital association has been developing databases in conjunction with the state health department. The hospital association has been following the issue in behalf of its hospitals but has not developed specific products or workbooks for its members.

For more information, contact Ms. Peg O'Keefe, Colorado Hospital Association, 2140 South Holly Street, Denver, Colorado 80222. Call (303) 758-1630.

Connecticut

The Connecticut Hospital Association has developed a statewide database of health indicators and other data pulled from various sources, including CHIME, which stands for Connecticut Health Institute Management Exchange, a hospital-based in-patient database that the association owns, from records of the Connecticut State Department of Health, from Medicaid, and from other sources. The association has just compiled the information and disseminated it to all of its members. The data are available on a statewide basis, and the hospital will run special analyses for individual locations for a fee. The association has begun a pilot program in which the association is working with a hospital that is the sole provider in a single hospital community. The association's role is to provide technical expertise so the community group the hospital is spearheading can develop a community health plan. There is no state requirement that hospitals conduct community health assessments, and one is not expected in the future.

For more information call Mr. Vin Prota, vice president, Connecticut Hospital Association, 110 Barnes Road, P.O. Box 90, Wallingford, Connecticut 06492-0090. Call (203) 265-7611.

Delaware

As of April 1995, there was no legislative requirement that hospitals conduct community health needs assessments or community service plans. The hospital association had discussed joining with the state medical society to develop a statewide process in which all its hospitals would join; however, the association decided not to implement this process. Instead, the association will work with hospitals on an individual basis to provide needed resources in this area. The precise parameters of the resources to be provided are at present unclear.

For more information, contact Mr. Joe Letnaunchyn, chief executive officer, Delaware Hospital Association, 1280 S. Governor's Avenue, Dover, DE 19904-4802. Call (302) 674-2853.

District of Columbia

In the face of overwhelming problems here, there is little formal needs assessment in progress; the needs are quite obvious. Hospitals are trying simply to survive. One-third of the people are below the poverty line, and

150,000 are on Medicaid, and in some hospitals, 18 percent of their patients unfunded. And no hospital in the District of Columbia is showing a profit. All run community clinics, community outreach services, public health clinics, mobile vans, and other services to try to deal with problems that are overwhelming. Because of the city's serious budget crisis, hospitals are downsizing, cutting back services, and laying off employees.

For more information, contact Holly Constant, District of Columbia Hospital Association, 1250 Eye Street, N.W., Suite 700, Washington, D.C. 20005-3992. Call (202) 682-1581.

Florida

Florida shows a range of interest. About 10 or 12 hospitals have gone quite far. The association, acting as a catalyst, has facilitated community groups coming together. Several hospitals are conducting health needs assessments as a group, and many others are moving in that direction but haven't gone that far yet. At present there is no legislative requirement. Hospitals are undertaking needs assessments to show their responsibility in the community and to show that they deserve their tax-exempt status. The hospital association sees itself as a catalyst in the process. It helps the individual hospital find out how to do it and who is doing it. They do not have anyone on staff, however, to act as a consultant to local hospitals.

For more information, contact Mr. Pat Haynes, senior vice president, Florida Hospital Association, 307 Park Lane Circle, P.O. Box 531107, Orlando, FL 32853. Call (407) 841-6230.

Georgia

There has been activity in Georgia, although I don't have precise numbers. Accredited hospitals are required by the JCAHO to do assessments, and others have done so, as well. The Georgia Hospital Association has a staff person who has been working with rural hospitals, which, in conjunction with their communities, conduct community health needs assessments. Each community appoints a community encourager, who pulls together a local healthcare council. The GHA staff person works as a consultant to train the encourager and to facilitate the process. He or she works with them to develop a multifaceted assessment, then pulls together the plan. Community health needs assessments are not mandated in Georgia now, and there is no evidence of any immediate move to do so.

For more information, contact Mr. Jeff Hill, coordinator of Community Assessment, Georgia Hospital Association, 1675 Terrell Mill Road, Marietta, Georgia 30067. Call (404) 955-0324.

Hawaii

The association has been talking about community health assessment but is in only the early stages. The state health planning and development office has been doing assessments island by island. It has done "the big island" Hawaii and Kauai, but we would be looking to supplement their data, because the data are often out of date and take a long time to produce. Hospitals aren't doing it on their own, and the association is still in the talking stages.

For more information, contact Mr. David Douglas, director for Health Care Information and Legislation, Healthcare Association of Hawaii, 932 Ward Avenue, Suite 430, Honolulu, HI 96814-2126. Call (808) 521-8961.

Idaho

There is a lot of activity in the field of health needs assessment in Idaho. In Twin Falls, for example, the community conducted a broad-ranging community health needs assessment and identified teenage driver-related accidents as a priority. Investigators identified one of the major problems was teens not receiving enough training during driver training, and they developed a way for kids to get added training via some sort of video game. In Boise, planners identified biking and use of helmets as major problems. The hospital association works to provide resources to hospitals interested in conducting health needs assessments but does not have a specific initiative in the field.

For more information, contact Ms. Bonnie Haines, senior vice president, Idaho Hospital Association, 802 West Bannock Street, Suite 500, P.O. Box 1278, Boise, Idaho 83701. Call (208) 338-5100

Illinois

No mandate exists in Illinois for community health assessment, but indications of interest are shown by increased hiring of people in those positions at the system and local hospital level. The hospital association, in conjunction with the state health department, is developing data on health statistics. The association has plans to develop initiatives more fully in the future, though it has not moved very far along in the process yet.

For more information, contact Ms. Nancy Krier, vice president of Professional and Clinical Affairs, Illinois Hospital and Health Systems Association, Center for Health Affairs, 1151 E. Warrensville Road, Naperville, Illinois 60566-7015. Call (708) 505-7777.

Indiana

A law, passed in 1994, mandates community service plans from about 64 voluntary not-for-profit hospitals in Indiana. The response has been mixed. A few hospitals have been conducting community health assessments for some time, but most still see it as obligatory. Though county-owned hospitals are not required to submit plans to the state, many are complying voluntarily. The hospital association has been encouraging hospitals to conduct assessments. Often the media will ask county hospitals for their plans; and, if a hospital does not have one, the media may portray the hospital negatively. The association has run a series of seminars and educational programs informing hospitals of the requirements of the law and walking them through the process. The association's staff will also meet with local hospitals to answer any questions concerning the law. However, the association has not produced a manual describing the process, and it does not have an in-house consultant dedicated to helping hospitals work through the process. Staff will answer questions and provide access to services of VHA or AHA, and it does not maintain lists of "endorsed" consultants. A major initiative has been undertaken through a joint project, consisting of the major hospitals in partnership with the state department of health. A spokesman for the association thinks that the other cities may follow suit in the near future.

For more information, contact Mr. Bob Mohr, executive director, Indiana Hospital Association, One American Square, P.O. Box 82063, Indianapolis, Indiana 46282. Call (317) 633-4870.

Iowa

The hospital association has just released information quantifying the benefits hospitals bring to their communities, plus a report on the economic value to their environments. According to a spokesperson, the association has not specifically focused on community health needs assessment, although it is looking at a number of options. According to the association, the driving force in Iowa is a simple desire to devise better ways of delivering care. The association is evaluating the kinds of services needed in the process.

For more information, contact Mr. Greg Boattenhamer, vice president of Communications, Iowa Hospital Association, 100 E. Grand Avenue, Suite 100, Des Moines, Iowa 50309. Call (515) 288-1955. Jan Jensen is executive vice president.

Kansas

There is no legislative mandate in Kansas, and it does not appear likely that there will be. The Kansas Department of Health and Environment, in conjunction with the Office of Local and Rural Health and the Kansas Hospital Association, worked in partnership to develop a series of workbooks given to each member hospital in March 1995. The workbooks walk readers through the process and provide some county-level data to assist users in the process. The workbooks contain health resources, morbidity, mortality, child health, census, and other data. The association will provide some resources but does not have a consultant on staff to assist users to work through the process. The CHAP process is reviewed in Chapter Seven. According to an association spokesperson, the hospitals were pleased to receive the information, but there was not a strong mandate to act.

For more information, contact Ms. Jerry Fried, data coordinator, Kansas Hospital Association, 1263 Topeka Avenue, P.O. Box 2308, Topeka, Kansas 66601-2308. Call (913) 233-7436.

Kentucky

No strong interest in community health needs assessments exists at the state level. Some hospitals may be interested, but, if so, interest has not reached the state association. The legislature in Kentucky meets every other year, and there is strong evidence that much of the healthcare reforms passed in 1994 will be repealed in 1996. If any interest is developing at the state level, nothing will happen until 1996 at the earliest.

For more information contact Ms. Peggy Ray, senior administration and assistant for Health Care Standards, Kentucky Hospital Association, 1302 Clear Spring Trace, P.O. Box 24163, Louisville, Kentucky 40024. Call (502) 426-6220.

Maine

As of December 1994, about two-thirds of the hospitals in Maine have done some sort of community health needs assessments. Most had constructed a demographic profile of their communities, but many of them have also looked at behavioral risk factors, health resource inventories, and utilization patterns; and some have gotten to the analysis stage, intervention planning. A few have been involved with PATCH for some time. The Maine Hospital Association is developing resources to help member hospitals in conducting community health needs assessments. These may include the following: (1) a set of guiding principles showing how hospitals should structure their assessments, how to define the community, and other issues; (2) a resource file of survey results and copies of questionnaires and instruments that hospitals have used in their assessments; (3) a list of consultants who have experience in the field; and (4) a listing of community health goals selected from *Healthy Maine 2000*. As of this date, the state of Maine has not required hospitals to conduct community assessments.

For further information on community health needs assessments in Maine, contact Ms. Kathleen Stuchiner, information services manager, Maine Hospital Association, 150 Capitol Street, Augusta, Maine 04330. Call (207) 622-4794.

Maryland

A spokesperson for the Maryland Hospital Association estimates that more than half of Maryland's 53 hospitals have conducted community health needs assessments. Many of them, as well, have been participating in an association-sponsored population health status assessment based on hospital discharge statistics. Community health needs assessments efforts in Maryland are driven by a desire to develop better relationships with communities and by a realization that, as the medical service delivery system restructures, the needs assessments will become key. The association is working to encourage and facilitate the process of community health needs assessments, but it has not developed materials or a guide. The association is developing an educational planning session to help hospitals develop partnerships with communities.

For more information, contact Ms. Nancy Fiedler, senior vice president for Communications, 1301 York Road, Maryland Hospital Association, Lutherville, Maryland 21093. Call (410) 321-6200.

Massachusetts

About one-half of the hospitals in Massachusetts have done community health needs assessments. There seems to be a consensus among hospitals, forged in part by the efforts of the hospital association, that the first step in responding to community needs is to know what they are. The level of investigation by hospitals varies considerably, though. Many have had a community advisory board for some time, and they have used that vehicle. Others have done comprehensive needs assessments, surveying business leaders, politicians, the general public, and other stakeholder groups and have put it together effectively. Almost all hospitals have used federal and state data sources to get at health indicators. The Massachusetts Hospital Association has had community benefit assessment as a key focus since 1991. The association runs seminars and other educational programs about various aspects of community benefits and how to do analysis. The association conducts and publishes the results from an annual survey to help members catalog what they are doing and to use in discussing healthcare issues with the legislature. Community health assessments are not mandated in Massachusetts; however, the attorney general's office has issued a set of guidelines and has placed public pressure on hospitals to comply. The hospital association does not maintain any data, or any endorsed consultant. Rather, it acts in a supportive role, providing access to resources and serving as an informal consultant with trustees, administrators, and others in hospitals to assist in specific aspects of community health assessment. The hospital association also sponsors a networking group and can put hospitals in touch with other hospitals that have done work in the area. The association has some literature on conducting community health needs assessments, but it has never put together any kind of kit.

For further information, call Allison Schneider, vice president of Communication, Massachusetts Hospital Association, 5 New England Executive Park, Burlington, Massachusetts 01803. Call (617) 272-8000.

Michigan

There appears to have been a lot of activity in Michigan, funded primarily by money from the Kellogg Foundation and by revenues from a tobacco tax. The state health department has pumped revenues from a tobacco tax into every local health jurisdiction to support community health assessment. The local health departments are not required to do health assessment, but if they wish money from the state, they must do so. Though the legislation targets the local health department, the local hospitals have become involved as well. More recently, the Kellogg Foundation funded community health assessment activities in a number of areas: in the Upper Peninsula, in three multicounty rural sites, and in several urban sites. In these areas the foundation has developed partnerships with communities in an effort to bring about long-term improvement in community health. There are no legal mandates in Michigan, although, in order to take advantage of revenues from the tobacco tax, communities are expected to undertake community health needs assessments.

For more information, contact Ms. Donna Strugar-Fritch, director of Rural Health Project, Michigan Healthcare Institute, Michigan Health Hospital Association, 6215 West St. Joseph Highway, Lansing, MI 48917. Call (517) 323-3443.

Minnesota

There is a lot of activity on a number of levels in Minnesota. Minnesota has 49 community health boards covering 87 counties. Some counties are covered by several boards, other boards serve several counties. The health boards, loosely related to the state department of health, conduct, according to guidelines laid down by the state, needs assessments every four years, and develop a four-year plan, which is updated every two years. Hospitals become involved in these plans because they are community institutions. They have been uneven partners in the process, in some communities becoming closely involved, in other areas only peripherally so. The state hospital association hopes they will get more involved. Private entities, such as insurance companies and employers, have also become involved in the process and have pressured local hospitals and communities to forge partnerships with the public sector. Regional coordinating boards, each constituting a cross-section of stakeholders, have served as effective mechanisms for bringing various stakeholders to the table. HMOs have been required to address a variety of specified public health issues, to look at those issues, and then, through action plans, to tell them how they are going to serve the population in those areas. No hammer is attached to it, but it is designed as a means for getting those plans to the table with local community health boards.

For further information, contact Melanie Soucheray, advocacy coordinator, Health Care Reform, Minnesota Hospital Association, 2221 University

Office Plaza SE, Suite #425, Minneapolis, Minnesota 55414. Call (612) 331-5571.

Missouri

The hospital association, in partnership with the state department of health, has developed a process described under the acronym CHART, which stands for Community Health Assessment Resource Team. Assisted by consultants, the team has developed an extensive manual designed to help communities pull together an assessment. The CHART team also will provide technical assistance to communities in implementing the CHART process. The process was "kicked off" on February 3, 1995, at eight sites in Missouri. The hospital association also has consultants that people can hire for a fee. The hospital association did not provide a copy for me to review.

For further information, contact Ms. Julie Simpson-Burris, Missouri Hospital Association, 4712 Country Club Drive, Jefferson City, Missouri 65109-4544. Call (314) 893-3700.

Montana

Community health needs assessments are not required by the legislature. The big issues in Montana were Medicaid and managed care reforms, which will be implemented here for physical health, mental health, and worker's compensation. Montana is just starting to see some interest in managed care, which is causing hospitals to do some more discussion locally on how to respond to it. These developments are encouraging more of them to do needs assessments locally. A number of local hospitals have begun to talk about hospital networks by region and need to do community health assessment not of just a community but of a region. The hospital association has been involved with a couple of regions on their network developments. The association has facilitated hospitals in contracting with consultants. It has no one on staff but has relied on outside expertise. In fact, the association distributed a request for proposals, for consultants on behalf of member hospitals.

For more information, contact Mr. Dick Brown, senior vice president, Montana Hospital Association, 1720 Ninth Avenue, P.O. Box 5119, Helena, Montana 59604. Call (406) 442-1911.

Nebraska

No legislation is pending in Nebraska. The hospital association has its strategic agenda for 1995 to focus on community health needs assessments. There has not been a large amount of activity in this area to date; however, hospitals are beginning to talk more seriously about it. The association will be looking for a consulting firm to assist it with developing community health needs assessments on behalf of its hospitals.

For more information, contact Mr. John Roberts, Nebraska Association for Hospitals and Health Systems, 1640 L Street, Suite D, Lincoln, Nebraska 68508-2509. Call (402) 476-0141.

Nevada

Nothing formal is going on in Nevada. There is certainly no legislative mandate, and the state hospital association does not provide ongoing assistance or consultation for hospitals in community health needs assessments. The association runs educational programs for its members, but it has no formal mechanism to help hospitals implement community health needs assessments. Individual hospitals are undertaking whatever initiatives or activities they wish to address about various health needs in their communities.

For more information, contact Hanria Holden, executive vice president, Nevada Hospital Association, 4600 Kletze Lane, Suite A-108, Reno, Nevada 89502.

New Hampshire

Efforts in New Hampshire seem to be driven largely from two sources. One thrust comes out of the Department of Health Policy and Management in the School of Health and Human Services at the University of New Hampshire. The second major initiative comes from the Dartmouth–Hitchkock Medical Center, which is spearheading community health needs assessments on behalf of its network of hospitals and group practices throughout New Hampshire, part of Vermont, and northern Massachusetts.

For more information, contact Mr. Jim Steaton, director of Membership and Development, New England Health Care Assembly, 125 Technology Drive, Durham, New Hampshire 03824-4724. Call (603) 862-1903.

New Jersey

New Jersey is quite active in conducting community health needs assessments. The association has been working on this since 1993. The association met with a spectrum of individuals: representatives of the New Jersey Department of Health, the state medical society, physicians, VHA, member hospital representatives, and others to develop a resource guide to help hospitals understand and conduct community health needs assessments. The association developed a comprehensive resource document and a video explaining how to do it, what sources to use, what data should be collected, how to store the data, and included several survey instruments. With the assistance of a consulting firm, the association is running five pilot projects in New Jersey. The association is also developing county health profiles of all counties, based on demographic and other data. The association is currently working toward having health-related data online and available through the Internet statewide. Rather than a response to the demand of individual hospitals, however, the activities of the association have been driven by a desire to encourage hospitals into the process. While member hospitals have been complimentary and receptive to the information, it is not clear about the extent of their interest in the process.

For more information, contact Ms. Valerie Sellers, vice president of Health Planning, The New Jersey Hospital Association, 760 Alexander Road, Princeton, New Jersey 08543. Call (609) 275-4261.

New York

All hospitals are required by law to develop community service plans. The statute as written excludes for-profit hospitals; but, since there are few of them, the law applies to virtually every hospital. That law, which expires December 31, 1995, is part of a prospective hospital reimbursement legislation passed periodically, and it has been in place since the late 1980s. At first hospitals were reluctant and saw it as an additional mandate. Now, while some are still lukewarm, others have found that it is a good strategic planning mechanism for them. Some have taken it very seriously and committed the time to do true needs assessments. Overall, hospitals are complying with it. Many are finding that, with managed care intensifying in the state due to mandatory Medicaid managed care law, community needs data are critical. Now that the requirement is coming up for renewal,

it is unclear if the requirement will be continued. The Healthcare Association of New York takes the position that it should be maintained, but that
the time period should be altered to every two or three years. As of April
1995, discussion about the requirement was just beginning. Also coming
under debate is the question of whether HMOs and other managed care
organizations should be required to do so as well. If hospitals are required
to improve the health status of the community, perhaps HMOs also should
be asked to do so. It appears likely that the requirement will be continued,
though perhaps less frequently. However, some argue that, if New York's
medical service delivery system becomes market-based, health needs
assessment should be incorporated into the strategic planning function
and no longer be required.

For more information, contact Mr. Paul Rulison, executuve director of
Hospital Trustees, Healthcare Association of New York State, 74 North
Pearl Street, Albany, New York 12207. Call (518) 431-7600.

North Carolina

There is quite a bit of activity going on here, basically on three fronts. One
effort stems from a governor's task force convened in the early 1990s, stim-
ulated by public health officials in North Carolina to develop programs at the
community level. Developed were local task forces and 22 active task forces.
Hospitals and communities across the state are encouraged to undertake
community health assessments and address the major needs in the community. Under the program, communities identify their primary health needs,
select a few of them, and develop a strategy for addressing them. Since 1974,
health departments have been conducting community health assessments
every two years; and, in many areas of the state, hospitals are teaming up
with their local health departments and other community groups to conduct
needs assessments. Hospitals work sometimes in partnership, sometimes
alone. Many of these have been funded by the Duke Endowment. The
hospital association has developed close relationships both with Sun Health
and with the state department of health. They have not developed a notebook
of their own, but they have arranged with Sun Health to make their workbook available to hospitals across the country. They have put on educational
programs and act as a resource for hospitals working through the process.
The workbook was not made available to me for review.

For more information, contact Ms. Ellen MacMillan, group vice president for Member Services, North Carolina Hospital Association, P.O. Box
80428, Raleigh, North Carolina 27623-0428. Call (919) 677-2400.

North Dakota

Hospitals have been quite active here. According to the preliminary results of a survey conducted by the North Dakota Hospital Association, 20 out of 50 member hospitals have either done an assessment or are in the process of conducting one. The interest has been generated by the hospitals themselves. Some analyses have been in depth. In Fargo, for example, the assessment was conducted by a community coalition consisting of hospitals, schools, and other community groups. An effort in Grand Forks apparently has also been quite wide-ranging. Smaller communities, too, such as Grafton, have done rather comprehensive efforts. Most of the groups conducting the assessments used resources in their communities, and they pooled expertise from universities, the local departments of health, or the state Office of Rural Health. In addition, hospitals that have done community assessments have provided information and assistance to hospitals considering doing them. The North Dakota Hospital Association has worked informally with the hospitals in North Dakota. The association runs seminars and educational programs on community benefits, but it does not have a dedicated consultant on staff, nor does it provide a workbook to local hospitals. Rather, the association places interested individuals in contact with appropriate resources as needed. Community health assessments are not mandated in North Dakota.

For more information, contact Ms. Nancy Willis, vice president of Communication, North Dakota Hospital Association, 1120 College Drive, P.O. Box 7340, Bismarck, North Dakota 55807-7340. Call (701) 224-9732.

Ohio

Ohio does not require community health needs assessments. The Ohio Hospital Association is developing a product with a statewide database, which will enable communities to use data more easily. Data will be county DRG data and age by sex will compare data for counties to the state for 1990 and 1993. This may be helpful retrospectively; however, it does not appear that the product as now envisioned will provide current data. The product will be available to members for a fee. Hospitals have shown some interest in conducting them, and a number of hospitals have teamed up to do them in conjunction with local community leaders. It is not clear, though, how intense it is at this point.

For more information, contact Ms. Karen Houk, Ohio Hospital Association, 155 E. Broad Street, Columbus, Ohio 43215. Call (614) 221-7614.

Oklahoma

Not a lot of activity exists in Oklahoma. Some hospitals have engaged in their own studies, utilizing consultants or their own staff; however, the hospital association apparently has little input into these activities. There is no legislative requirement for voluntary hospitals to conduct needs assessments.

For more information, contact Mr. Keith E. Calvert, vice president Risk Management, Oklahoma Hospital Association, 4000 Lincoln Boulevard, Oklahoma City, Oklahoma 73105. Call (405) 427-9537.

Pennsylvania

Community health needs assessments are not mandated in Pennsylvania, but the state hospital association has promoted community needs assessments for its hospitals. Through its shared services program, the association has developed a handbook, available for a charge, which can assist local hospitals in working through the process. An association spokesperson estimates that the interest in community health assessment is growing in Pennsylvania, and that 25 percent of hospitals are either in the process of conducting them or have done so. The association provides "initial hand-holding" and access to resources for hospitals in conducting assessments, and it has staff available to give advice and to link hospitals with people who can assist them. But the association does not have a consultant on staff specifically dedicated to working with community assessments. The association also provides a list of "endorsed" consultants to whom they will refer interested hospitals.

For more information, contact Mr. John Hope, vice president Communication Services, Hospital Association of Pennsylvania, 4750 Lindle Road, P.O. Box 8600, Harrisburg, PA 17105-8600. Call (717) 561-5335.

Tennessee

At present there is no state mandate, but there is some interest in it because of the pressure placed by TennCare, Tennessee's new Medicaid management program. TennCare has created some upheavals and alerted the state about the need to focus on community health issues. Most of the activity is centered in urban areas, where hospitals are better staffed. Hospitals in Memphis, Knoxville, and Nashville are beginning to develop communitywide health information sharing networks, largely under the pressure of large employers. An initiative in Knoxville began as a way for hospitals to track child abuse cases among those families that appear to be "emergency room shopping." Nashville and Memphis are also active, driven largely by the pressure of large employers. The hospital association is beginning to focus on community health needs assessments, particularly with rural hospitals. It has run a workshop on community health needs assessments and plans to sponsor a networking group. The association thinks its initial activity will be with rural hospitals, which are not as well staffed.

For more information, contact Bill Ives, vice president, Information Services, Tennessee Hospital Association, Interstate Boulevard, S., Nashville, Tennessee 37210. Call (615) 256-8240.

Texas

The state of Texas requires community health assessments of not-for-profit hospitals and of hospitals that have a high proportion of Medicaid patients. These account for slightly more than half of Texas's 480 hospitals. The hospital association has produced a manual to help hospitals work their way through the process and runs seminars and educational programs to train hospitals in conducting health needs assessments. However, it does not provide consulting or other technical assistance to hospitals involved in the process. There appears to be considerable interest among the hospitals themselves. A spokesman for the Texas Hospital Association guessed that many hospitals would be doing community health assessments even if they weren't mandated by the state.

For more information, contact Mr. Jon Hilsabeck, Texas Hospital Association, 6225 U.S. Highway 290 E., P.O. Box 15587, Austin, Texas 78761-5587. Call (512) 465-1000.

Vermont

Some activity exists in a couple of communities: Rutland and Brattleboro. In the latter, the effort has sprung from the public health department there, though the hospital is participating in the process. There has also been an effort in the Franklin/Grand Isle area in northwestern Vermont, where community organizations banded together and completed an assessment. The association serves as a resource center for hospitals that have questions about conducting a project. It maintains a library of resources and links hospitals with other resources, such as the American Hospital Association's resource center. Some of the staff have provided informal consulting to a number of groups thinking about launching their assessments. Community health needs assessments are not mandated by the state of Vermont.

For more information, contact Peter Holman, vice president for Planning and Regulatory Affairs, Vermont Hospital Association, 148 Main Street, Montpelier, Vermont 05603. Call (802) 223-3461.

Virginia

Activity in Virginia is uneven. Some hospitals have done quite a lot and have partnered with many different organizations. Others have not addressed the issue yet. All the hospital association would share with me is that it is currently collecting information on specific hospitals. More specific information was not available.

For more information, contact Ms. Barbara Brown, director of Clinical Information Services, Virginia Hospital Association, P.O. Box 31394, Richmond, Virginia 23294. Call (804) 747-8600.

Washington

There appears to be significant interest and activity in the state of Washington. I don't have any statistics, but interest is flowing from two sources. First, the newly approved Public Health Improvement Plan has pressured local health departments to conduct community health needs assessments. Hospitals have become involved in the process at two levels: the state hospital association was represented on the task force that developed the initiative at the state level, and local hospitals have become involved in the efforts of local health offices to develop community health assessments. A second driving force has been the spread of managed care and capitated markets. Hospitals are trying to find out where they fit in the new capitated environments.

For more information, contact Ms. Katharine Sanders, coordinator, Community Health Networks, Washington Health Foundation, 300 Elliott Avenue West, Suite 300, Seattle, Washington 98119-4118. Call (206) 285-6355, ext 509.

Wisconsin

The Wisconsin Hospital Association has been actively promoting health needs assessments in the state. The association has developed a guide, based on elements taken from various processes reviewed in this book. It has distributed the guide to each member hospital, and it is conducting a series of workshops to encourage hospitals to team up with their communities. The guide has been reviewed in Chapter Seven. A second impetus for community health needs assessments lies in the local departments of health, which, under state statute, must conduct health needs assessments in communities. The state department of health has conducted training sessions for local health departments, and local hospitals have been encouraged to work with them. A third driving force in some communities has been local groups that have initiated health planning and have involved hospitals in the process. Though some hospitals have embraced the process, the reaction of most hospitals has been lukewarm. Many chief executive officers have seen it as important, but buried it in their list of priorities by "more important operational issues."

For more information, contact Ms. Marsha Borling, director of Patient Care Services, Wisconsin Hospital Association, 5720 Odana Road, Madison, Wisconsin 53719. Call (608) 274-1820.

Wyoming

Interest in Wyoming is in developing an office of rural health. This office would assist local communities and hospitals in developing health needs assessments. However, the office was not sufficiently funded to accomplish these goals. Hospitals in Wyoming apparently have shown some interest in community health needs assessments, but most of them haven't done it. Testing the tax-exempt status of hospitals has come up in the legislature but has not progressed very far.

For more information, contact Mr. Dan Perdue, vice president, Governmental Relations, Wyoming Hospital Association, 2005 Warren Avenue, P.O. Box 5539, Cheyenne, WY 82003. Call (307) 632-9344.

Conclusions

By now, you and I have taken quite a trip together. I hope that you have had as much fun reading this book as I have had writing it, although, at the end, I must admit I am ready to give it up.

Together, we have learned the following things. At the beginning we saw how the paradigm shift has brought healthcare providers into a new world of expectations. Providers now are expected to take responsibility for the overall health of the people that live in the communities they serve, rather than the people just inside their buildings. Then we saw that new assumptions will require hospital managers to expand their vision of health, to assess the primary needs of their communities, and to redesign the delivery of medical services in such a way that they contribute to the overall health of the community, and that they restructure their activities to act as a catalyst to groups in the community. Then we briefly viewed the health promotion process and showed how the assessment process fits within it; we defined community health needs assessments; and we reviewed the basic components of an assessment: constructing a community health status profile, collecting secondary information where necessary, devising an assessment plan, conducting a community leader survey, conducting a health-related behavior survey, developing goals and objectives based on the outcome of the research, revising our plan and implementing specific projects, and reevaluating the process and the outcomes of our efforts. Then, in the next few chapters, we saw the specific results generated from six community health needs assessments and reviewed a number of models of them. Toward the end of the book, we learned about research, and we learned some pointers about research and how to avoid some of the major pitfalls. Then we took a brief ride through the assessment landscape. Throughout this book I have ardently encouraged you to use a research firm where research is called for.

THE GOAL IS IMPROVEMENT

I hope that you heed the call of this book and broaden your vision toward a wider view of health and healthcare. Once this is done, you will find new partners in your community, and new gains will be made in improving the relationships between your hospital and the community. Strong efforts in this regard can only improve the overall health of the community and bring a better life for everyone.

Index

About the Author

Tim is an experienced healthcare consultant with more than 25 years of experience in research and analysis. He earned his Ph.D. from the University of Wisconsin–Madison in 1980. He was on the staff of the University from 1972 to 1982, and he worked for the State of Wisconsin's Department of Development in 1982 and 1983.

Tim began his involvement in market research in 1982, and began to work with healthcare organizations in 1984. He headed up National Research Services, Inc., from 1982 to 1989; was Vice President with Heron Associates of Greenwood, Indiana, from 1989 to 1991; directed business development and research for Indiana University's Center for Entrepreneurship and Innovation from 1991 to 1992; and he is currently Vice President of Marketing Research in Health Care at Young & Associates where he directs the firm's healthcare services group.

Tim has conducted over 250 qualitative and quantitative studies for hospitals, managed care organizations, and insurance companies across the country. His expertise includes moderating focus groups, administering telephone and mailed surveys, conducting executive interviews, and experience with secondary research and analysis. His studies have included community health needs assessment, consumer opinion surveys, and market studies to address the behaviors, preferences, attitudes, and opinions of significant stakeholder groups. Most recently, he has conducted research studies in Bakersfield, California; Ames, Iowa; Osage Beach, Missouri; Pittsburgh, Pennsylvania; and Fairmont, Minnesota.

Tim's primary professional goal is to develop long-term relationships with clients to help them meet the challenges facing their hospitals, their communities, and the healthcare system of our nation. He values strong personal relationships, growth, creativity, helpfulness, honesty and directness in working with others, and having fun.

Tim resides in Madison, Wisconsin with his wife and family. He has three children, aged 16, 17 and 21, and a granddaughter aged 2. His hobbies include photography, traveling, playing chamber music, crossword puzzles, writing poetry, and following the University of Wisconsin's basketball, football, and hockey teams.